FIVE MINUTE
STRETCH

FIVE MINUTE
STRETCH

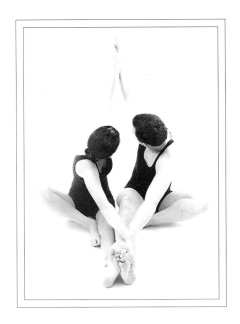

Robert Thé

Virgin

First published in 1996 by
Virgin Books,
an imprint of Virgin Publishing Ltd
332 Ladbroke Grove,
London W10 5AH

Copyright © 1996 Robert Thé/Virgin
Publishing Ltd

A catalogue record for this book is
available from the British Library

ISBN: 0 7535 0075 2

Printed and bound in Great Britain
by Butler & Tanner Ltd,
Frome and London

Photography: Katie Tueton
Models: Jennifer Long,
Martin Bannister, Oscar Rowley,
Kassie Landau, Charlie Reading

Make-up: Nadira Persaud

For Virgin Publishing: Carolyn Price

Design: Paul Kime

This book is dedicated to my mother

Special thanks also go to:

Miguel Buss
Felicity & Amber Jay
Smita Joshi
Paul Kime
Petrushka
Carolyn Price
Rosa
Maxine & Oscar Rowley
Rokiah Yahman
Kit-Ford Young
Steve Young

Thank you all for your continued support and encouragement.

Robert Thé
London
February 1996

C O N T E N T S

INTRODUCTION

There once lived a man who trained fleas. As soon as they were born, he carefully separated them and put them in their individual glass jars. He put enough food in each jar for them to survive and sealed them with metal lids which had holes in them so that they could breathe. Soon they began to grow larger and larger and, fleas being fleas, began to flex their muscles. Unfortunately, every time they jumped the young fleas would hit the lid. And after several jumps, the fleas learnt to gauge the height of the jump exactly so that they wouldn't hit the lid and damage themselves.

In due course, the man removed the tops of the jars. At last freedom was possible! However, the fleas had already learnt to jump only so high and no higher. And that's how the freedom that was theirs by birthright and only a short hop away was lost forever.

Although most of us might smile wryly at these creatures' lack of vision, this story has much to teach us about the danger of self-imposed limitation and how easy it is to lose sight of our full potential.

We are born with tissues, muscles, joints and limbs that breathe possibility and freedom. Yet something happens over the course of the years, so that from an almost infinite repertoire, our movements become few, predictable and boring.

It's not too hard to see how this begins. As children we are rarely encouraged to express ourselves physically. Instead, we have to learn to sit still in dull classrooms under commands not to fidget or yawn at a time when our bodies are bursting with life and the desire for movement. To make matters worse, when we most need to release tension and stagnant energy – after long periods of sitting down – we are told not to stretch because it is considered rude!

It is hardly surprising, then, that in a culture that discourages listening and responding to the body's needs and wants the body starts to shut down or go to sleep. After all, how likely is it that you would keep trying to make conversation if you were with someone who never listened to a word you said?

Far too often the cost of growing up and adapting to the demands of a mainly sedentary society is that our bodies become distant relatives. We know that they exist and hear from them from time to time, but theirs is a strange country and we understand the language of computers, cars, and tax forms far better than the strange dialect that our body speaks.

Bewitched by the demands of the outside world which constantly clamour for our attention, we lose connection with the process of change and dialogue that occurs within our body on a daily basis. As this happens, the body responds by forgetting its true potential for unrestricted movement, convincing itself that the limited and repetitive patterns it experiences are the norm.

However, as muscles become congested and tissues denser, it becomes all too easy for the body to begin a slow spiral of decay: the flow of blood which brings life-giving oxygen to our cells slows to a trickle as it struggles to reach the tissues and muscles, the lymph fluid which clears debris and toxins becomes trapped and unable to escape from our cells, and our life energy, vital for keeping our body systems balanced, becomes cut off and stagnates. Our body's efficiency begins to diminish and as our muscles become progressively more congested and we begin to lose our flexibility, this can have a surprising effect on our thinking, which can become similarly sluggish, slow, and predictable over time.

An additional result of losing connection with our bodies is that it becomes harder to hear and respond quickly to various warning signals the body gives out when it is in distress. For example, how many people have worked at a desk for hours on end, their attention fully absorbed by a computer screen, only to discover to their surprise when they finish that they have a raging headache and back pain which seems to have come from nowhere? However, it's not as if our body suddenly sends an SOS as soon as we have finished our task. Rather, with our attention completely focused on the outside world, there was no one left to notice the maydays, emergency flares, and ship sinking slowly beneath the waves.

One of the best ways of reversing this process of limitation and decline and learning instead how to listen to the body's needs is through stretching. Far from being the domain of yogis, contortionists and professional athletes, stretching is for everyday people leading busy everyday lives who want to remain loose and supple and is one of the most natural and intuitive behaviours – just watch a cat or dog as it stretches and realigns itself several times during the course of a day.

The specific benefits

A vital part of remaining healthy involves keeping the muscles flexible and the body generally supple. By stretching we can reduce any stiffness and tension that builds up during the day, releasing it before it can begin to exert any negative effect, and help to develop and maintain our maximum range of movement.

Stretching can also develop toned muscles and stamina, allowing us to become stronger. In addition, done prior to strenuous physical activity it can help to protect the body from injury and so is an essential part of any exercise programme.

One of the byproducts of stretching can be a general increase in vitality. This is because as muscles relax and joints become supple the energy channels in the body open up, releasing stagnant energy and allowing it to travel freely throughout the body, creating a sense of being truly alive. And while stretching can provide us with a burst of energy when we most need it, it can also help us to unwind from all the daily

stresses and tensions, silencing our restless minds, centring us, aligning our physical and mental energy, and leaving us feeling rejuvenated, calm and alert.

However, despite these benefits, stretching is sometimes seen as something of a chore: something most people feel they ought to do but never quite get round to. This is probably because of a general perception that stretching is physically demanding, requiring a lot of discipline in order to feel the benefits. With many traditional stretching approaches focusing purely on relaxing tight muscles and holding cheerless static positions for long periods, this perception is somewhat understandable.

But stretching is not only about becoming more flexible and having loose muscles. At its highest level, it is about reawakening the body through awareness and movement. With this focus, we don't have to stick to standard stretches: we can take any movement and by bringing awareness to the movement, we can turn it into a stretch. Through such gentle reminders, we can awaken the memories of past possibility, experience more space in our tissues, unlock our full potential and create room for our soul to play, create and grow.

So rather than focus only on developing flexibility, the emphasis in this book is on exploration, pleasure, movement, awareness and the discovery of new possibilities. This is why in these pages you will also find exercises derived from Tai Chi, Qi Gong, yoga, modern dance and massage which are not traditional stretches in the strict sense. However, they will help you to heighten your sensitivity and awareness and increase your enjoyment of the simplest movements.

The more regularly you listen to your own body, the quicker you will be able to hear changes that need to be addressed before they turn into limitations or physical discomfort. In addition, listening in this way enables you to fully inhabit every muscle, tissue and joint.

$\mathcal{H}$ow to use this book

This book is divided into three parts. The first is devoted to stretching for one and two people, from the moment we get up to the time we close our eyes. There are sections on preparing mind, body and soul for the day ahead, recharging at work, keeping relaxed and supple while travelling, gearing up for exercise and sport and finally winding down and preparing for sleep.

The second section focuses on the early and later stages of life. The earlier we begin as children, the more likely it is that our bodies will retain their suppleness and vitality throughout life. It's never too late to start stretching, however, and as we enter our later years, regular stretching and movement can help to maintain and increase our youthfulness and well-being.

The final section, the appendix, lists all the exercises contained in the book according to which area of the body they are designed to stretch. Consult this if there is an area of your body you particularly want to open and become more flexible.

To obtain the best results from this book:

- Read through each exercise before attempting it
- Ensure that the environment is as warm as possible, as this helps the muscles to remain relaxed
- The looser your clothing, the better
- Try to avoid eating heavily before doing any stretching
- Don't force any movement – be gentle with your body
- Start with small movements, gradually becoming larger
- Slow, deep breathing is the key to success, breathing out as you feel the stretch
- Consciously relax into each stretch
- Don't bounce at the end of a stretch

- Stop if you notice any sharp pain or anything untoward
- Hold as long as the stretch is comfortable for you
- The more regularly you stretch, the more you will notice the benefits: flexibility comes with time.

There is no set way to work through this book. I recommend that you use it on an as-and-when basis and allow it to grow into your life – that way you'll absorb the information at your own pace, and it's more likely to have a deeper and longer-lasting effect.

These exercises are designed as an invitation for you to explore the potential of your own body: suggestions to help you remember the freedom which is your birthright. You should use the ideas and images in this book as springboards and create your own personal stretches.

The most important thing to remember as you begin to move and stretch is not the duration of each exercise but your state of mind. You will get more out of each exercise if you approach it by becoming aware of how you are moving and what it feels like, rather than mechanically doing it and thinking about what you're going to have for dinner later. Think of each five minute exercise as your own sanctuary away from the pressure and demands of the outside world – a time for you to listen and acknowledge yourself in the here and now.

I hope that you enjoy using this book for many years to come and that you get everyone around you involved and regularly experiencing the power and benefits of Five Minute Stretch. So dive in, enjoy and here's to your health!

Five Minute Stretch has been designed so that it is suitable for everyone. However, there are certain circumstances when stretching should be avoided.

These are when you:

- are ill
- have had any recent accidents or injuries
- have had any recent surgery
- have experienced any recent muscle or joint damage
- have any major physical problems

Do bear in mind that these are general guidelines only: in certain circumstances, stretching can be instrumental in helping you return to health. For example, after certain muscle or joint injuries, encouraging the body gently to begin moving again can help restore full mobility. The most important thing is to use your judgement, and if you are in any doubt please consult your medical practitioner.

When working with a partner, please check that they have no condition which would prevent them from receiving a Five Minute Stretch. To obtain the maximum benefit from working with them, please be sensitive to their comfort and ask for feedback to ensure that you are responsive to their needs.

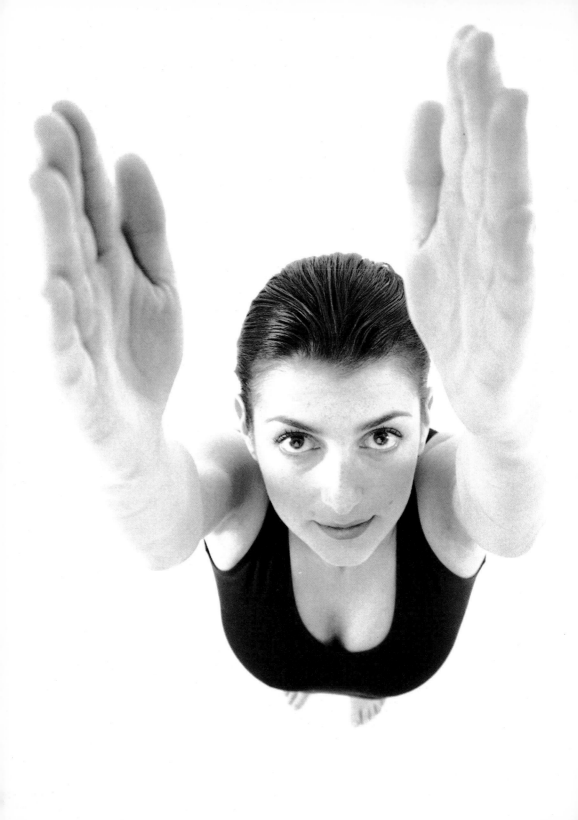

Greeting The Day

The way we wake up and begin the morning can make an enormous difference to how we feel and react during the course of the day. So it is worth starting in a positive way.

When my cat, Petrushka, wakes up she always has a really good stretch before even thinking about the other important things in life such as eating and chasing birds. Human beings, on the other hand, tend to alternate between lingering in bed as long as possible or launching themselves into several must-do activities before rushing out of the house for their next destination, usually still half asleep and invariably late.

During the night the body often remains in the same position for long periods and many of us feel a little stiff and low in energy when we wake up. After a while we might feel awake mentally, but our body still hasn't had a chance to wake up fully and we can feel sluggish and under par for a large part of the day. Stretching is a great way for the body to switch on, ready for the day ahead: joints can be realigned, muscles stimulated, and blood and energy encouraged to flow freely throughout the whole body.

So if you want a 100 per cent mind-body-spirit kind of day, include some of these simple stretches in your morning routine. From then on it's all systems go and ready for take off!

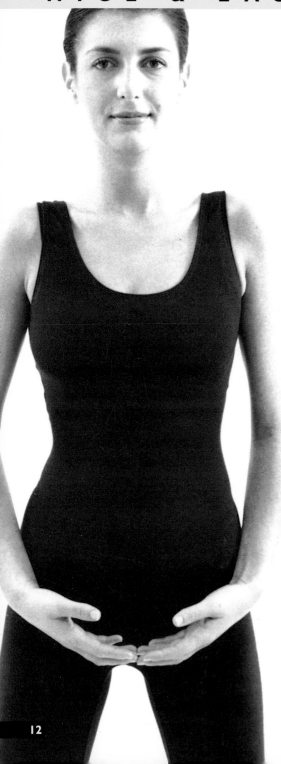

𝒯he last thing that I want to be faced with on first waking up are complex and challenging stretches, and I can imagine that's how you feel too. That's why I've created these stretches so that they're easy to do even when you're not fully awake.

These simple and gentle stretches are designed to loosen the body, especially the major joints, which can become stiff and stop energy from flowing freely in the body. When you stretch you might hear them click occasionally, which shows that stagnant energy is being released. This is a healthy sign, a sign of being truly alive, and of more energy being released into your life.

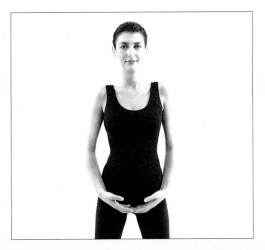

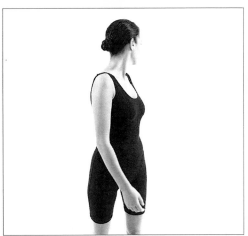

1 Begin by standing with your feet slightly apart and your hands by your belly. Bend your knees slightly and imagine that your head is connected to a hook in the sky, aligning and lifting it upwards. Breathe slowly and deeply into your navel area several times. This position will focus your energy and awareness.

2 Allow your arms and hands to hang loosely by your sides. Imagine them to be quite heavy and then start swinging from side to side slowly. Let your head follow the movement. This is a great move for loosening up the torso and improving the breathing.

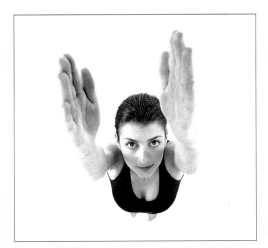

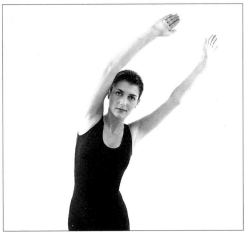

3 Straighten your legs, raise your arms as high as possible and stand on tiptoes.

4 Keeping your arms in the air, lower your heels to the ground and then gently stretch first to the left and then to the right several times. Then return to the initial stance and centre yourself once again.

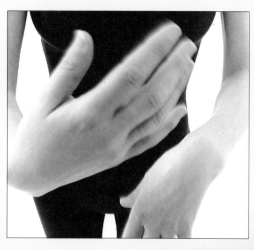

*I*f you've got out of bed and tried some gentle stretching but you still feel that your eyes are bleary, your brain has shut down and your main fire needs some stoking, it's definitely time to shake out them blues.

| Begin by shaking your wrists gently in front of you. Try shaking them together first and then in different directions. Maybe they are equally loose or perhaps one is a little stiffer than the other.

Using vibration, shaking or any other movement is a great way of kickstarting the day since it gives the body a chance to be activated and for stagnant energy to be cleared. Why not use music together with these moves since it'll get things moving and your juices flowing? Whoa! Whole lot of shakin' going on ...

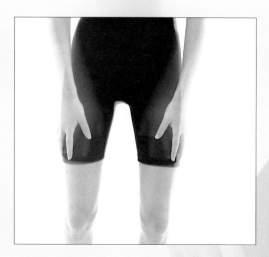

4 Next place your hands on the front of your thighs and start to vibrate them gently. Try also working the sides and backs of the thighs and then start shaking the whole leg. Don't forget the muscles in your bottom, too!

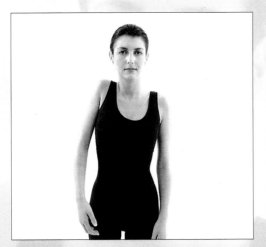

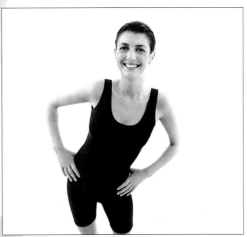

2 Then focus on your shoulders, moving them side to side, up and down, round and round. This can release dormant energy and feels good to do as well.

3 We spend so much time sitting that the pelvis can often become stiff, which can reduce our overall flexibility. Try to move your hips in as many different directions as possible.

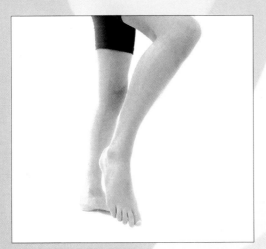

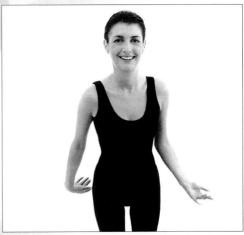

5 Lift one leg off the ground and then shake the ankle. If you can imagine any stress or tension falling out of your body as you do so and being absorbed by the ground, so much the better. Repeat with the other ankle.

6 Now the grand finale. Combine everything you've just done and shake your body all over. Let every part of you move, wobble and shake, and breathe out anything that you want to let go of as you begin a virgin day.

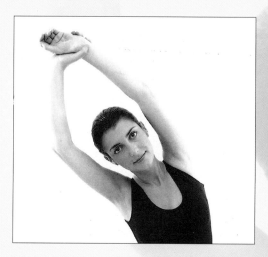

There is often a close connection between how free we are in our body and how we respond to life and the changes it brings. By discovering where we are restricted and taking appropriate steps to release these areas, we can often set in motion small changes that will reverberate through our life, opening up new possibilities.

I Stand with your feet apart and bring both hands together above your head. Grasp the wrist of one hand and allow the weight of the arm which is over your head to help you bend to the side. Come back to centre and repeat on the other side.

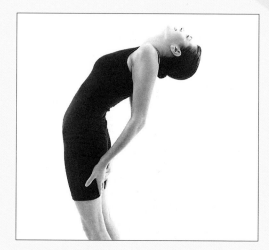

4 Now try a counterbalancing stretch. Stand with your feet apart and place your hands on the backs of the thighs. Push your pelvis forwards and bend backwards and walk your hands as far down your thighs as they will go.

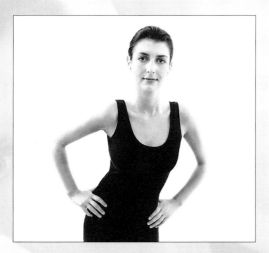

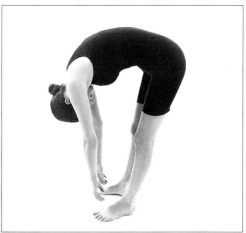

2 Place both hands on your hips and begin to rotate your hips in a clockwise direction. After a while, begin rotating them in the reverse direction and then from side to side.

3 Next allow your head and arms to hang loose and slowly begin to bend forward, leading with the head. Continue as far as is comfortable and no further. Then reverse your movements, with your head the last to straighten up.

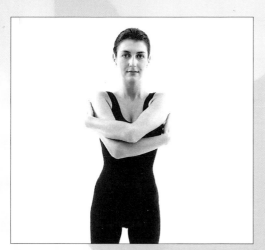

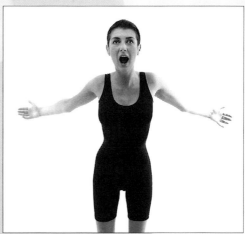

5 Come back upright, hug yourself, take a deep breath and make a loud sound as you fling your arms out to the sides.

6 Repeat several times and then place your hands by your navel and refocus yourself by breathing slowly.

*M*odern physics confirms what the ancients have always known: we and everything that surrounds us are made up of energy. Sometimes it is easily recognizable, like the heat of the sun or the force of an exploding volcano. Sometimes it is almost invisible, locked deep within as in a kilo of plutonium, and sometimes it is generated between individuals, in a sharp exchange or a moment of love. Energy can be sensed and felt. It may take time and practice before you can do it, but there is nothing like feeling your own energy, your life-force, coursing through your body. So why not try these stretches, experience them fully with your senses? Slow, beautiful and vibrantly calm, they are a good way to centre yourself for the day.

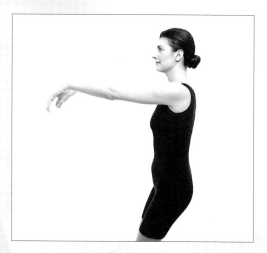

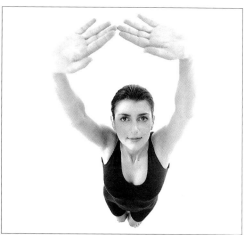

1 Take a slow breath and raise your arms in front, imagining you are drawing the energy of the earth into your body. As you breathe out, bring your arms out to your sides and then lower them.

2 Next raise both arms straight up above your head, palm upwards as if you were supporting the sky. This creates a good stretch along the arms and opens your energy channels, helping all your internal organs to function better.

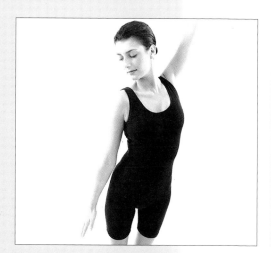

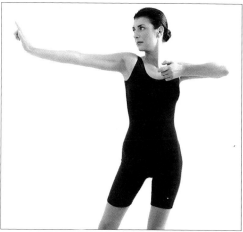

3 Then bring one of your hands down while stretching as high as possible with the other. Let your gaze follow the descending hand, then let it go back up and repeat with the other hand.

4 Point your right foot outwards and bring your right arm out to the side with the palm facing outwards and the index finger pointing upwards. Look at your right hand and bring your left hand back as if you were drawing a bowstring.

$\mathcal{E}$veryone knows that mornings can sometimes be something of an obstacle course, with even your nearest and dearest seeming to conspire to make you late. However, by including someone else in your morning stretch routine, you can bring a dash of fun into getting up and preparing for the day.

These exercises are taken from Japanese massage techniques and are a great way to loosen tight muscles, encourage the body to become open and bring a smile to your lips. So why not give them a try?

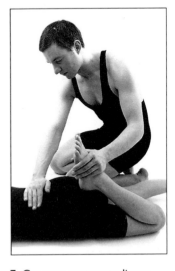

❙ Get your partner to lie on their stomach. Place one hand on the bony area of their lower back, and with the other hold one foot and bring the leg slowly in towards the buttocks. As they breathe out, bring it closer but stop if they feel uncomfortable. Then stretch it to the side of the buttock. Repeat with the other leg.

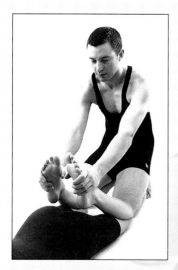 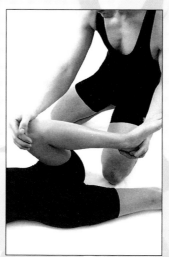 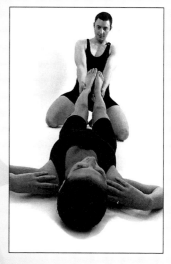

2 Then move round to their feet and bring both legs up towards their buttocks. Your partner should feel a good stretch down the front of their legs. To deepen the stretch, cross their legs and bring them in again.

3 Now ask your partner to turn over. Put your hand under one foot, put the other hand on their knee and bend their leg into their body. Then start to take their whole leg into a rotation. Try different directions, if you want.

4 Next take both feet and, leaning back gently, take their legs into a nice long stretch. Then go round to your partner's head, squat down and do the same for their arms. Let your partner have a few moments to rest and enjoy the feeling of wellbeing they will have.

LISTEN & STRETCH

*H*ere are a few suggestions which you might like to explore with a partner. These stretches work best when both people are listening to each other, not trying to compete, not going beyond what is comfortable. In addition, you might find that one of you is a little more flexible than the other. If this is so, show respect for the other person's physical limits and pace the stretch accordingly.

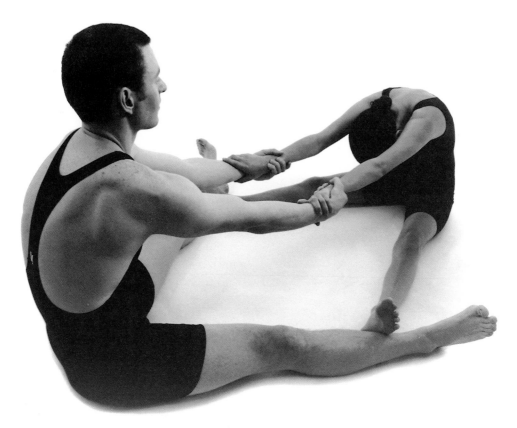

■ Sit on the floor with your legs apart, facing your partner. Allow your feet to touch the inside of their legs, then lean across and grasp each other's wrists and take turns to gently pull one another.

Slowly begin to pull each other in a seesaw fashion. As you become more used to the movement, increase its depth until you can experience a good stretch along the back.

2 Sit facing your partner with your legs straight in front of you. Bend your knees slightly so that the soles of the feet touch. Then bend forward and grasp your partner's wrists. Grasping firmly, press against both feet and lift both legs into the air at once. Hold for as long as possible, then lower and release.

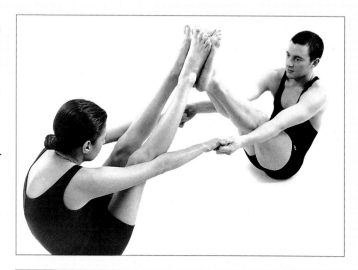

3 Sit side by side with adjacent legs outstretched and touching. Then tuck the outside foot on the inside thigh. Bend to look at each other and use the outside arm to clasp the sole of each other's foot. Stretch the other arm up with the palms pressed together and look up at the hands. This should create a noticeable stretch around the spine and the torso. Hold for a few breaths and change sides.

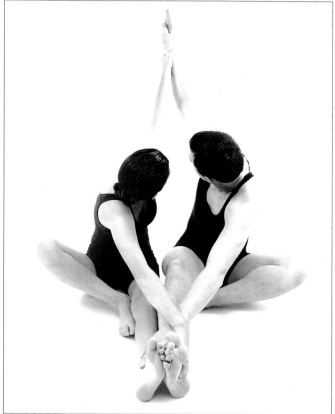

Here are some dynamic yoga poses which have been adapted for two people. They are challenging and will require some balancing and co-ordination on your part, but if you are willing to be patient and to experiment these stretches will be very rewarding. After finishing, you should feel more toned, focused, grounded and highly charged, ready for an action-packed day.

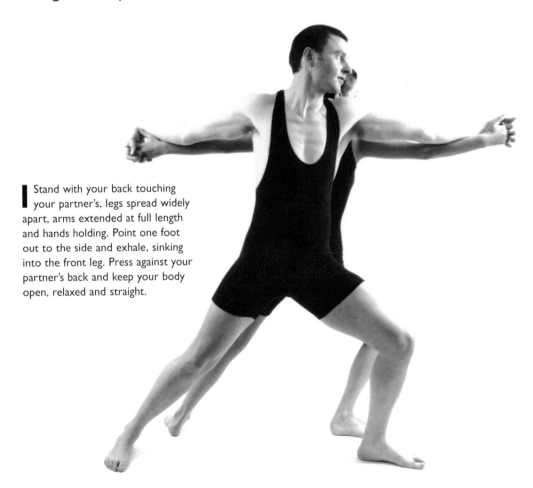

1 Stand with your back touching your partner's, legs spread widely apart, arms extended at full length and hands holding. Point one foot out to the side and exhale, sinking into the front leg. Press against your partner's back and keep your body open, relaxed and straight.

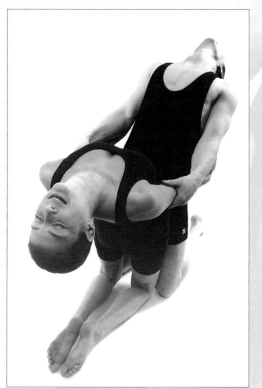

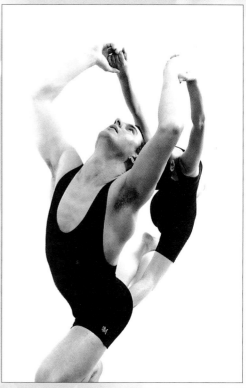

2 Kneel in front of each other with the front of your thighs touching. Grasp each other by the arm or elbow and slowly arch backwards as far as is comfortable.

3 This stretch is excellent for the thighs, pelvis, shoulders and back. Stand with your backs to each other, well apart. Bend the left knee and take the leg back so that the leg is as flat as possible on the floor. Sink your hips down and bring your arms over your head, arching your back so that you can hold your partner's hands.

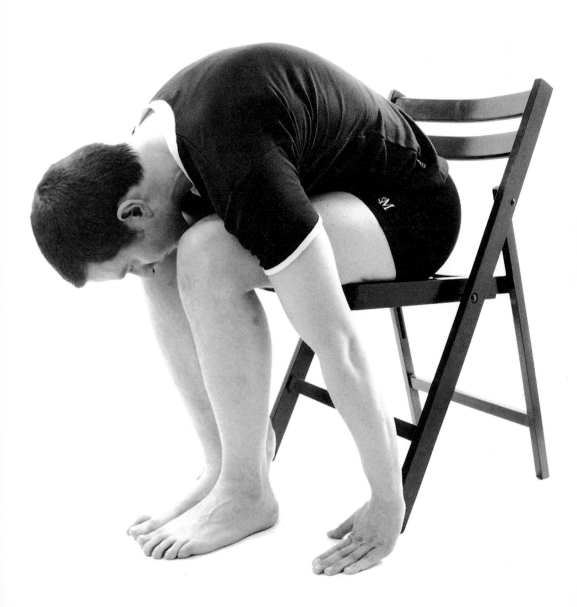

While You Earn

Increasing pressure to perform under larger workloads and cope with new technology has turned the modern workplace into something of a battlefield, where the main casualty is our body.

Lest you think I am exaggerating, statistics show that millions of working days are lost from work-related stress and physical injuries such as back pain. This scenario is not just confined to this country but is taking place right across the world, making it a problem of global dimensions and adding weight to the general belief that working can be dangerous to your health!

Our bodies evolved through movement and they expect physical freedom. Yet in many ways, the workplace of today represents a denial of this basic biological heritage, with jobs designed so that we spend hours or even the whole day in the same position, rooted to the same small area.

This has the effect of shutting the body down, which can mean that we ignore signs of discomfort and physical distress until they literally explode into our awareness as a severe headache, a stiff shoulder or agonizing back pain. You can reverse this process and become more in tune with the messages your body constantly sends you by regularly taking time out to stretch while you earn and inject some movement and life back into the day.

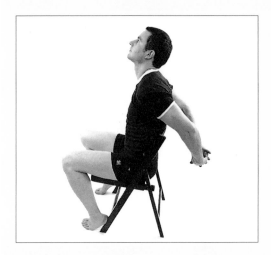

Studies show that people who don't take time out during the working day and push themselves with disregard for the body's needs are actually less efficient than those who do. Far from being a luxury, taking short regular breaks to refresh yourself physically during the day is essential. So next time you do take time out, enjoy the thought that although it may look as if you are doing nothing for ten minutes, you are, in fact, working hard to make your organization more effective and productive!

In a sitting position, clasp your hands behind your back, straighten your arms, bring your hands down, gently bring your shoulders back and feel your chest open and expand.

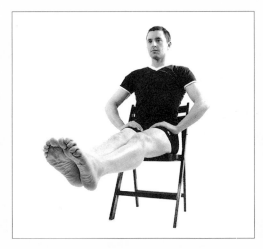

4 Stick both feet straight out and feel the legs stretch along their entire length.

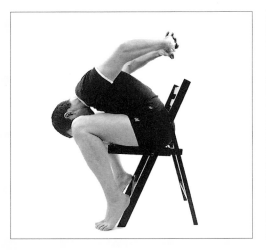

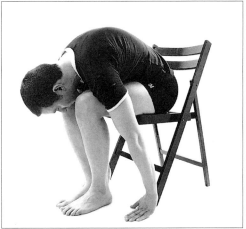

2 Still keeping your hands together, bend forward in your chair and bring them as far over as you can. This might seem quite tricky initially, but it will get easier and is great for releasing stiff shoulders.

3 Release your hands and, still bending forward, allow them to touch the floor. If you are really supple, you can see how far you can reach behind your feet!

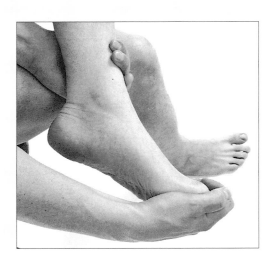

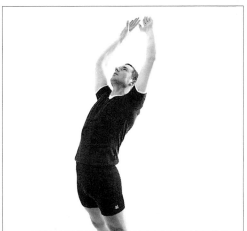

5 Put one leg down and place your other foot on top of the thigh. Wiggle your toes, creating a sense of space, and use your hand to rotate your ankle.

6 Finally, stand up, raise your hands above your head and lean back. This creates a strong stretch along the front of your body.

*M*odern working practices often involve repeating the same motion over and over again which can lead to a progressive loss of suppleness. Tense, stressed bodies are more susceptible to injury and the number of people who suffer from symptoms such as aching muscles, sore or swollen joints, has now reached epidemic proportions. If they are not caught in time, these symptoms of over-use can develop into much more serious conditions. Stretching regularly at work can help to break up any tension as it develops.

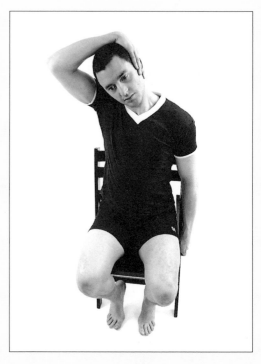

Place your right hand over your left ear and as you pull your head towards the right, push your left shoulder down. This creates a very powerful stretch. Then change hands.

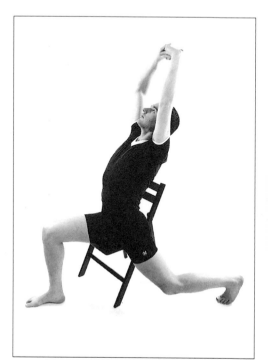

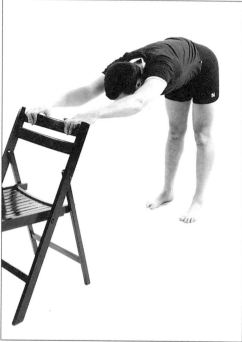

2 Sit diagonally on the corner of your chair and stretch your left leg out as far as you can behind you while raising your arms above your head and leaning back.

3 Stand a few feet away from the back of your chair. Placing your hands on it for support, slowly bend forwards and let the weight of your trunk create a stretch between your shoulders.

*A*mong ergonomists – professionals who are concerned with creating the best work environment for the human body – there is major discussion about what to do with the chair, with some demanding that we give up the attempt to improve on the basic design and recognize that the chair always has been and always will be a dangerous four-legged beast.

This sounds extreme but when you look at the effect the chair has on the body it makes more sense. Not only is sitting down for long periods far from ideal for the back, it also compresses the stomach, liver, spleen and kidneys, which can interfere with digestion.

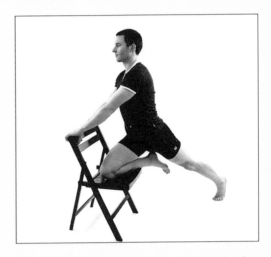

Place one knee on your chair with the other leg straight out to the side. Lean forward on to the knee to open and stretch the muscles on the top of the thigh.

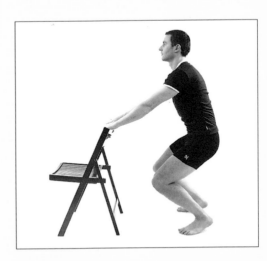

4 Keeping your arms out straight, gently bend your knees. Slowly increase how far you bend, and don't forget to breathe while you do this.

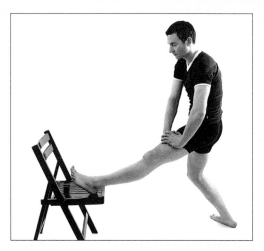

2 Next place the heel of your foot on the chair. This will straighten your leg and if your stance is quite wide you should feel a strong stretch in the hamstring muscles. You can vary this stretch by placing both hands on the tops of your thighs and bending your other leg.

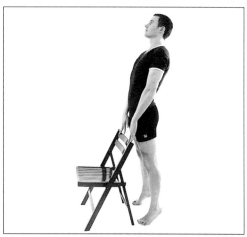

3 Stand away from the chair a little and use it as support as you raise yourself on tiptoes, noticing which muscles are being used in the process.

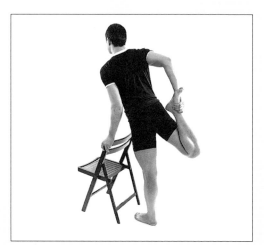

5 Keeping your left hand on the chair, bend your right leg behind you and grasp your right foot with your free hand. This will create a stretch all along the front of the right leg. If you lean back slightly, this stretch will extend along the front of your body. Repeat with the other leg.

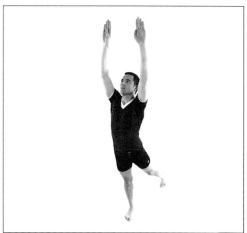

6 End with a full stretch. Standing on one leg, raise both arms up and away from your body and stretch your free leg behind you as far as you can. Repeat on the other side.

In Japan, the working day is often preceded by a communal stretch. This not only helps everyone to relax and limber up for the day, but also promotes a positive working environment and sense of team spirit.

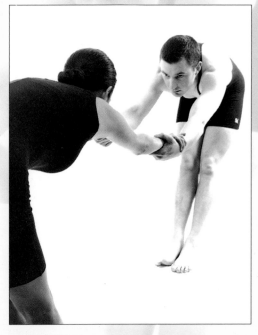

In sharp contrast to Eastern practice, which emphasizes co-operation within the group, we in the West are brought up to be fiercely proud of our individual achievements and

Stand opposite your partner. Keeping your legs straight and your feet together, bend forward and clasp your partner's wrists. Breathe out and lean into the stretch, allowing your pelvis to move back and your spine to lengthen.

competitive within group situations. Although this approach does have its merits, it does little to create a unified work environment. By taking stretch breaks with your work colleagues you can begin to build small bridges towards a co-operative and harmonious environment.

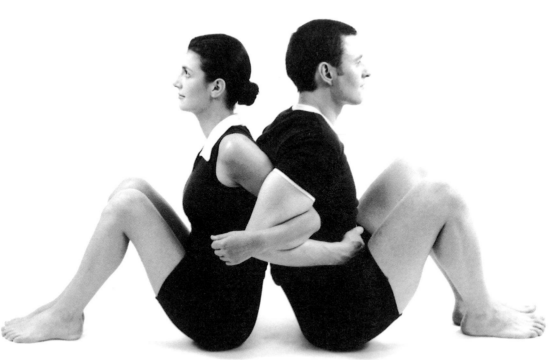

2 Sit back to back on the floor with your knees bent. Then lock your arms together at the elbows. Breathe in and as you exhale, push against the floor and one another in order to stand up. This can be pretty hilarious, so don't try to take it too seriously. Gently sit down again and repeat as often as desired.

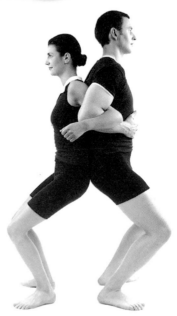

In the future, the companies that will thrive in a tough, competitive market place will be those that have invested in the wellbeing of their staff. Far from being an expensive luxury, employee healthcare is a priority which can determine productivity levels. So if anyone asks you what you are doing when you try these exercises with your colleagues, tell them you're 'improving the bottom line'. Who knows, they might even promote you!

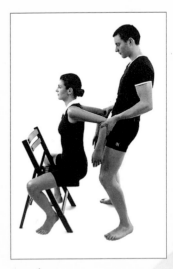

Slide your hands down to your partner's wrists. Bring your hands back up slowly, grasping their forearms just below the elbow.

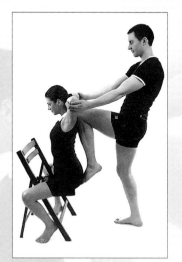

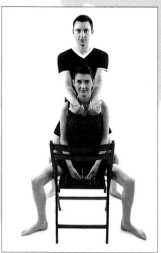

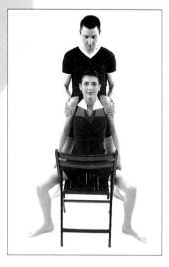

2 Next ask them to clasp their hands behind their head and place your front leg gently in the middle of their back. Ask them to take a slow, deep breath and pull their arms towards you. Lower their arms gently back down.

3 Place your forearms close to the base of their neck so that your elbows are parallel. Then bend your knees slightly and allow your body weight to compress the shoulder muscles. Release the pressure and repeat a few times, moving further along the shoulders each time.

4 Ask your partner to take a deep breath, grasp them firmly by the upper arms, raise their arms about 2 inches (5cm) and release your hands, letting their shoulders fall down. Repeat several times and conclude with light massage.

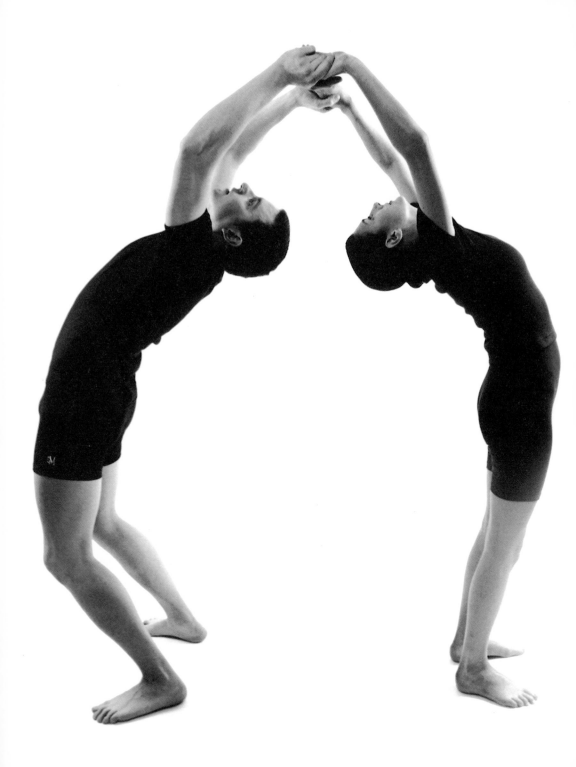

From A To B

How far we have come in a hundred years! Whereas at the turn of the century a journey between two main cities would have been a major excursion, these days we would hardly consider that a journey at all.

Today we take it for granted that we can board a plane and before long be touching down halfway across the world in an exotic country, with a different time zone, climate and customs. With travel so commonplace, hundreds of millions of people around the world are on the move, travelling to see friends and family, conduct business, move to new areas, look for work or simply take a holiday, and they are using a wide variety of transportation – cars, bikes, buses, trains, boats and planes – to get there.

However, as more people hit the trail, more time than ever is spent going from A to B – and no matter how glamorous the means of transport, there is no getting away from the fact that travelling often means remaining in the same position for several hours or even longer. This can take its toll and leave you feeling physically worse than when you first set out – so if you want to make the most of travelling, try some of the following stretches when you are next on the road.

I love visiting new places, meeting new people, discovering new cultures. However, being in transit can take its toll, and as someone who opted to travel around Europe on ludicrous 30-hour coach journeys and spent three days on board a packed Chinese train, I've experienced aches and pains in the most unlikely places. So if it feels as if you've got something resembling a dagger stuck between your shoulders, your neck has turned into a block of wood and your back doesn't believe the word relaxed exists, these exercises might help you go the distance.

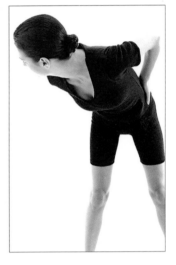

| Place your hands by your waist and lower back. Turn your upper body at an angle to the right and bend slightly to look down. Then allow the torso to travel to the opposite side in a smooth semi-circle, breathing slowly as you bend forward. Return to the centre, breathe in, lift your head and chest and look towards the front.

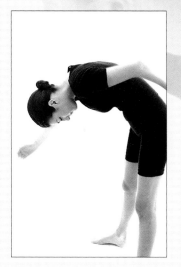

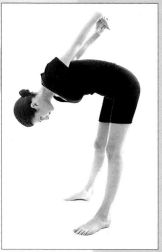

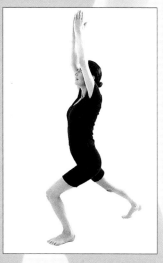

2 Bend forward and begin to roll and rotate your shoulders. This not only releases tension in this immediate area but also loosens the chest and aligns the spine.

3 Lock your hands behind your back, straighten your arms and slowly bend so that your head comes forward and your arms begin to rise. Allow them to come forward as far as possible and then slowly come back into an upright position. This relaxes the back muscles.

4 Adopt a lunge position with your left leg bent and your right leg straight behind you. Put your hands together and raise your arms straight up. Let your head drop back slightly and allow the front of your body to stay upright.

As anyone who drives knows, long-distance motoring can be exhausting. The twin challenges of paying constant attention to the road and the mechanics of driving – manoeuvring the steering wheel, using your feet to work the accelerator and brake, changing gear – can be particularly stressful and can leave you physically and mentally drained.

Stopping regularly during your journey to take care of yourself for a few minutes can make all the difference. It will help to clear your head, improve your concentration and awareness, and dispel any physical tension that has built up. Try it, and arrive in better shape.

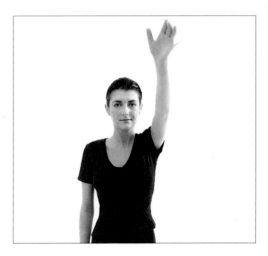

Start with some gentle arm circles which will help to relax the shoulders and stimulate circulation in the whole area.

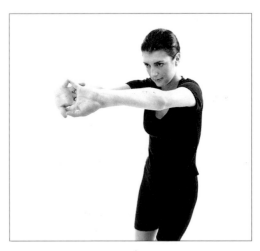

4 Bend your knees slightly and tuck your pelvis in. Interlock your fingers, palms turned outwards, and straighten your arms out as far as possible. You should feel the muscles relaxing between the shoulders as your upper back opens slowly.

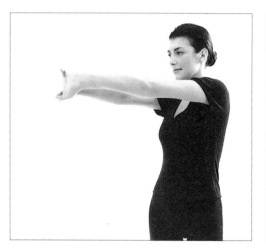

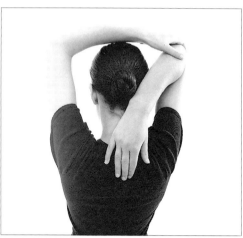

2 Then lock your hands together, invert them so that the palms are facing outwards and begin to swing your arms horizontally from side to side. You should notice a stretch along the back of the arm muscles.

3 Place your right arm behind your head so that your hand is at the top of your spine. Reach over with your left hand, grasp your right elbow and gently begin to pull towards the left. This will create a good stretch along the side of the chest, releasing built-up tension. Change hands and repeat.

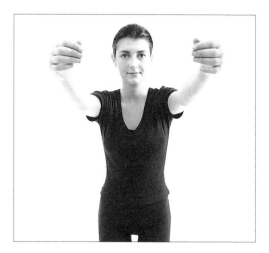

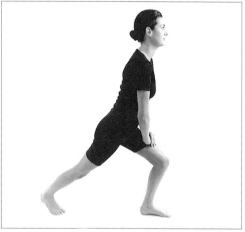

5 Bend your knees again and as you straighten them, throw your arms up in the air so that they come down as you bend your knees again. Repeat the move and develop a rhythm.

6 Extend your right foot backwards and place your left foot forwards, keeping your upper body straight. This should create a long stretch all the way down the front of your extended leg. Hold for a minute and then change legs and repeat.

*E*very year more people take to the air. Flying is now so popular that some airport executives publicly doubt whether they will be able to satisfy demand over the next few decades. With many airports already at maximum capacity, check-in queues becoming ever longer and departure lounges increasingly crowded, you're likely to be pretty stressed before the plane has even taxied to the runway. So if you are going to fly the world, remember to pack this book and try these exercises. They could be just the ticket!

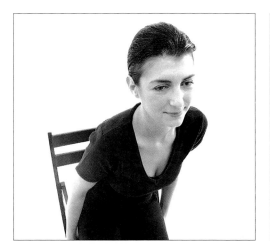

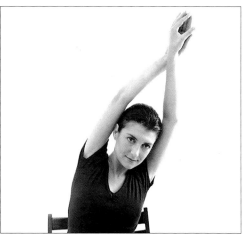

1 Slowly begin to rock from side to side on your seat and then allow the movement to evolve into wide circles. This will help to open up the lower back.

2 Raise your arms above your head and invert the hands so that the right hand is on the left and both palms are touching. If you lean first to one and then the other side you should feel a very strong stretch.

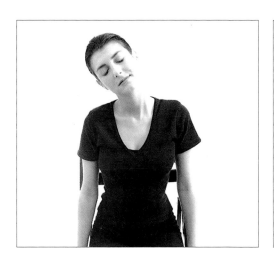

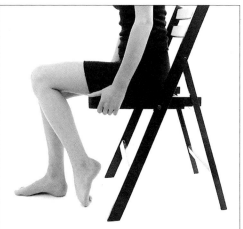

3 Next release any tension in your neck by bringing your head first to one side and then the other, then in slow circles and lastly turning it from side to side. Don't forget to change direction from time to time.

4 If you can kick off your shoes for this stretch, so much the better. Press your foot down, curling your toes underneath, and push it forward against the floor. This stretches the muscles in the foot and the front of the leg. Repeat with the other leg.

*H*aving someone stretch with you as you travel can be a great way of making the journey more enjoyable as you both release all the aches and tensions that have built up. If you take your time with these stretches, not only will you become aware of exactly where you need to open up and relax, but you'll also be amazed at how quickly the miles can be soothed away and the spirit fully refreshed. So let these stretches take the strain – and bon voyage!

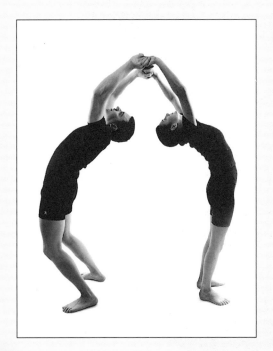

Stand back to back about 3 ft (1m) away from each other. Standing with your feet slightly apart, bring your arms overhead and join hands with your partner, then straighten your arms and start to arch back, leaning towards each other and breathing evenly throughout. This is a great stretch which lengthens the spine and loosens the back muscles.

2 Stand side by side with your feet apart and one foot touching your partner's. Hold hands and lunge towards the outside foot, stretching away from each other so that the inside of the torso is lengthened. Then twist away from each other and round the outside to face the back and take both arms over as far as is comfortable. Swop sides and repeat so that the other side receives a stretch too.

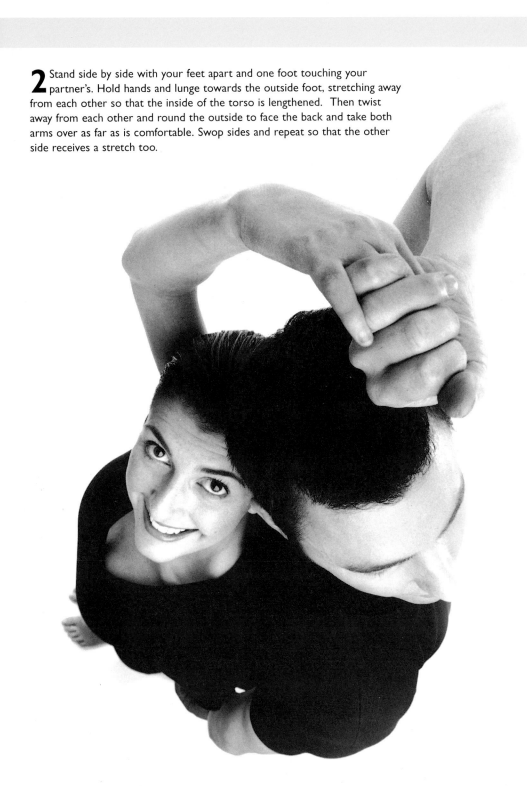

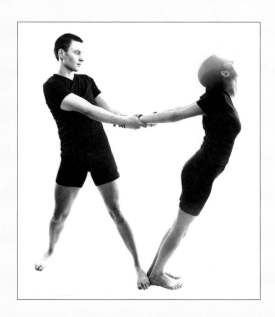

*J*ust between you and me, the chief advantage of travelling with another person is that not only do you have someone with you who can provide amusing conversation and company, they can also give you great massages and stretches. Mind you, they probably think the same thing about you, so I guess you'll have to take turns to exploit each other. While you decide who goes first, cast your eye over these suggestions and see if they take your fancy.

Note: Do not do exercise number 2 if you have a history of back complaints, and avoid doing this with anyone who is very different to you in size or weight.

Stand straight with your feet together and your heels against the outer edge of your partner's foot. Reach back and clasp wrists and then arch forward, pressing your feet into the ground. Your partner should support you as you lean forward, opening the hamstrings, expanding the chest, shoulders and back and lengthening the spine.

2 This is a great stretch if done properly. Stand with your back to your partner with your feet firmly on the ground. Then put your arms through theirs, support their bottom with the small of your back and bend over slightly, bringing them on to your back. You should both breathe calmly throughout. When the stretch is finished, lower your partner gently back on to the floor.

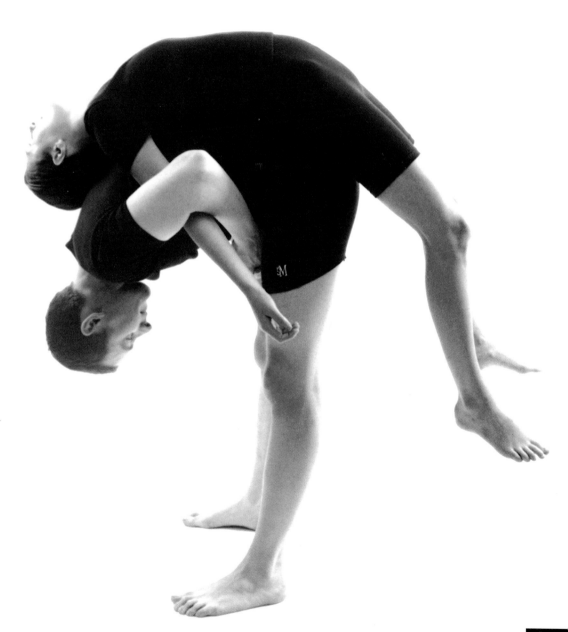

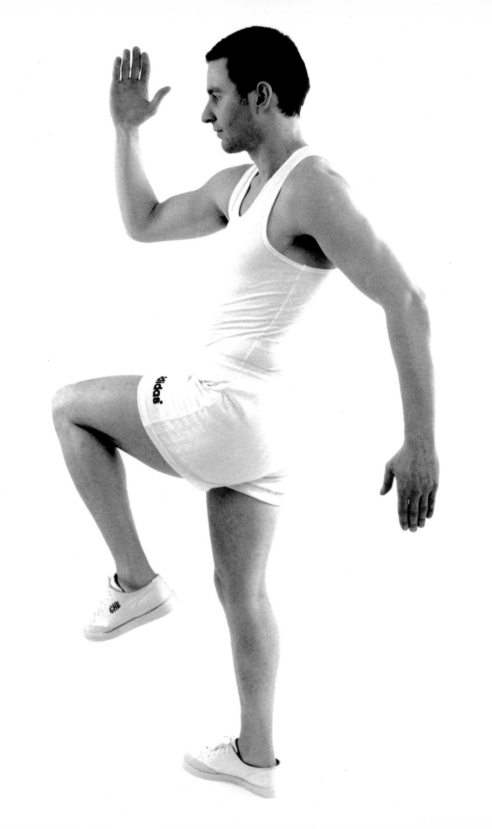

Everyone's A Winner

Stretching before you engage in any strenuous physical activity is very important. I used to be a keen rugby player at school and warming up and stretching prior to training or playing a match seemed a bit of a bore.

It wasn't until someone in the team had to be carried off the field with a torn muscle and our coach explained to us that it was probably because he had skipped the warm-up and stretch session that I realized there maybe was a point to preparing the body before 'the real action' after all.

Exercise and sport are meant to be beneficial, but if your body is not warmed up and taken through a series of stretches beforehand, not only is it totally unprepared for any demanding movements that might follow, making muscular injury a possibility, but with your muscles still tight your sporting performance can be drastically reduced and what should be enjoyable exercise becomes hard work instead, leaving you feeling worse than when you began.

So, regardless of whether you are already a professional or are just exercising or playing sport for your own health or pleasure, make sure you stretch at the beginning and you'll never lose in the end.

𝒯he first step in preparing for physical activity is warming up, which should come before any stretching. This involves waking the body up and allowing blood to begin to circulate throughout the entire body, particularly deep within the muscles. This increases their internal temperature, helping them to soften and relax, making stretching easier and preparing them for the physical demands of sport and exercise later on.

Although everyone agrees on the importance of warming up, few people realize how vital it is to have a cooling down period as well. This can help to stop muscles from tightening and contracting after physical exertion, release any tension or toxins that may have built up within them, help improve recovery time and prevent sore muscles the day after.

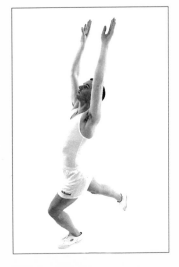

I Take a step forward with your left foot and breathe in as you bring your arms up high. Feel the stretch along your body as you breathe out. Bring your foot back and come back to a standing position. Take a deep breath and repeat with the other leg.

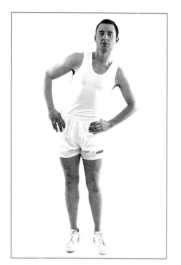 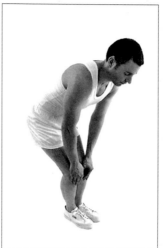 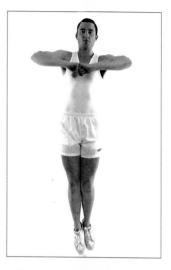

2 Next begin to rotate your hips in a clockwise direction. Increase the rotation gradually.

3 Then work with your knees. Stand with your feet together and hands on each knee and begin to move in small circles.

4 This should get your pulse going. Begin by placing your forearms parallel to your body and your fists facing each other. Then jump, twisting the lower part of your body to the left and bringing the upper part to the right. Then jump again, bringing the legs across to the right and the torso to the left. Repeat as many times as you need until you feel properly warmed up.

*O*nce you have warmed up, it is time to take your muscles and joints through a basic routine which will remind them of the possibility of movement. Doing this will not only help to loosen tight muscles even further, but will also improve your circulation.

Developing flexibility and becoming more relaxed before you exercise is the true foundation for physical fitness. Not only do individual muscles become more supple, alert and responsive, but muscle groups begin to work in harmony, allowing you to become more efficient and helping you to attain your true physical potential.

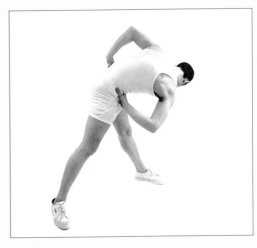

Place your hands on your hips. Leading with your right elbow, twist to the left and then repeat to the right with your left elbow.

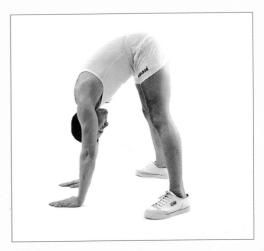

4 With legs apart and breathing slowly throughout, allow your body to bend forward until your hands are as near the floor as possible.

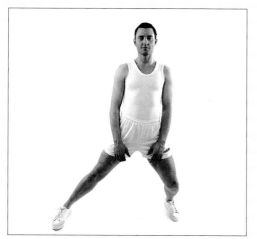

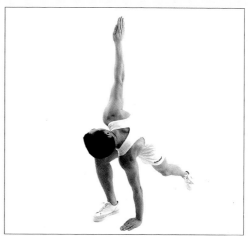

2 Then stand with your feet apart and bend your left knee slightly. This creates a stretch along the right inner thigh. Keep your upper body straight, hold for 30 seconds and then reverse legs.

3 Go into a lunge position and place your palm slowly on the ground. Raise the free hand vertically above your head and turn to look at it. This creates a deep stretch along the front of the body. Repeat on the other side.

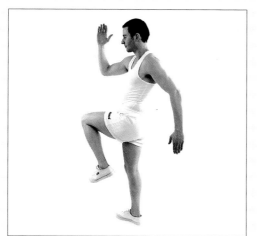

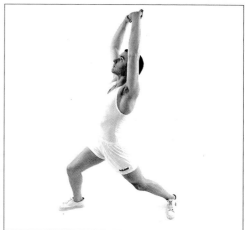

5 Stand with your feet slightly apart and arms hanging loose. Then bring your left leg up and across to the right and your right arm up and across to the left. Then repeat this cross-stretch with the other leg and arm.

6 Go into lunge position again and let your torso face the same direction as the foot pointing forwards. Bring your arms up above your head. Clasp your hands loosely and lean right back for a full stretch.

$\mathcal{W}$armed up? Feeling looser? Time then for some stretching to develop your range of movement, strengthen and tone your muscles, and focus your mind and body so that both react as one. This will enable you to enjoy your activity more, and provide you with freedom of movement, improved co-ordination, speed and stamina.

These stretches are mainly static stretches, where you gently take a muscle as far as it can go and then hold it for up to ten seconds. The muscle can then relax, which allows you to take it further. The longer you hold the stretch while breathing slowly, the greater the stretch you will experience.

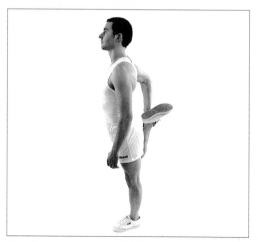

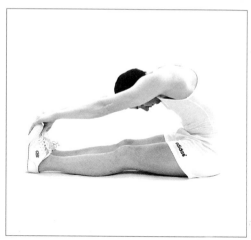

1 Standing up, bring your right leg back and grasp your ankle with your right hand. Bring your foot slowly towards your buttocks. You should feel a strong stretch along the front of your thigh. Repeat on the other side.

2 Sit down on the floor, legs straight in front of you, and slowly bend forward as far as you can, breathing out. This is particularly good for tight hamstrings and lower backs – but do be patient with yourself and take your time.

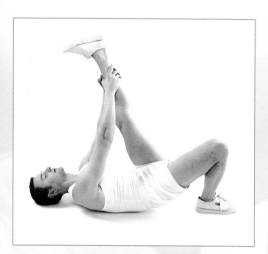

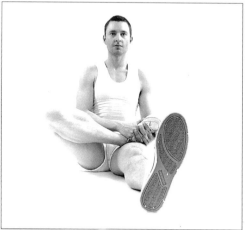

3 Lie on your back and bring your knees up slightly, then slowly bring one leg up and catch it with both your hands. Straighten it slowly, and as you do so you should feel a strong stretch along the hamstrings. Bring the leg as close to your chest as possible and repeat on the other side.

4 Sit up with both legs straight in front. Grasp one foot with both hands and slowly bring it in towards your belly as close as you can without causing any discomfort.

A LONG STRETCH

Although it might sometimes be tempting to bounce at the end of a stretch to push it further, this can actually do more harm than good. This form of stretching, called ballistic, used to be quite popular, but a bounce is registered by the brain as a muscle suddenly and unexpectedly being taken beyond its normal range of movement. The brain perceives this as dangerous and immediately sends a signal to the muscle concerned to tell it to contract – so while you are trying to relax and stretch a muscle, bouncing in fact triggers the reverse effect and can cause long-term damage. Static stretches may take a little longer and need a little patience, but they provide the longest stretch and get you there in the end.

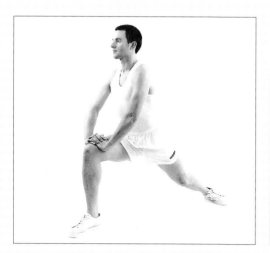

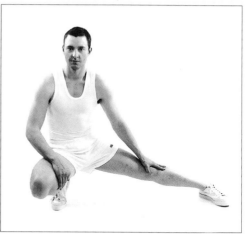

1 Point your right foot forward and bend the knee, then place both hands on top of your right thigh and allow your left leg to slide back as far as it can go. Then repeat on the other side.

2 With feet parallel and wide apart, bend the right knee and crouch down as low as possible. This will cause your left leg to straighten and you should feel a powerful stretch on the inside of your leg. Slowly transfer your weight to the other side.

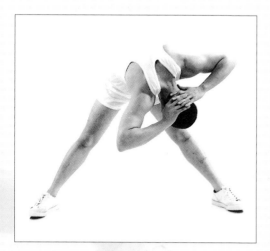

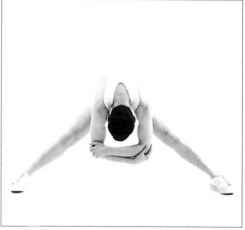

3 Feet wide apart again, put your hands behind your head and turn your upper body to the left. Slowly bend forward until you are looking at your right thigh. This is good for developing a flexible upper body.

4 Finally, increase the width of your stance and allow yourself to bend forward. Clasp each elbow and let your arms and head hang loosely. Hold and breathe slowly as the hamstrings experience a powerful stretch.

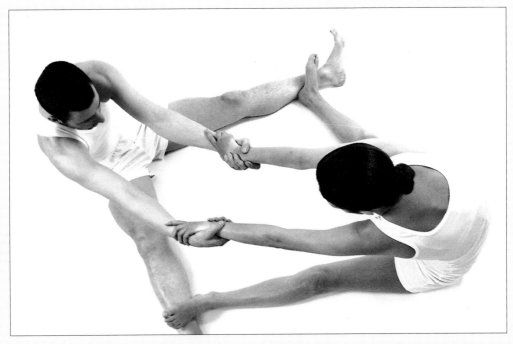

*S*tretching with another person can make limbering up for exercise or sport a real pleasure. Try these suggestions after each of you has warmed up on your own. Pulling together not only helps you to loosen up further than you thought possible but can also make for greater co-operation and teamwork.

Sit facing each other with legs wide apart. Place your feet against the inside of your partner's ankles, providing resistance. Then grasp your partner's wrists and gently begin to pull your partner forward. This will not only open the upper back but will also loosen the pelvis.

Take it gently, breathe throughout, work within your partner's limits and change over when ready. Another possibility is to set up a circular rhythm between the two of you, and slowly increase the size of the circle.

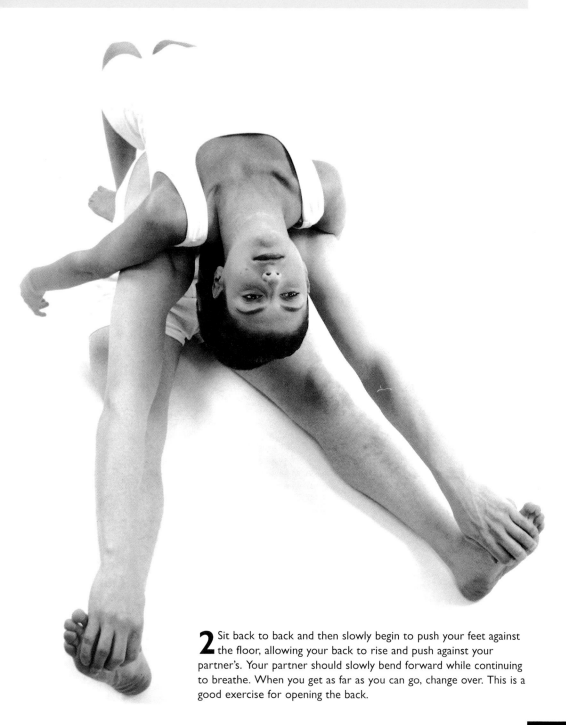

2 Sit back to back and then slowly begin to push your feet against the floor, allowing your back to rise and push against your partner's. Your partner should slowly bend forward while continuing to breathe. When you get as far as you can go, change over. This is a good exercise for opening the back.

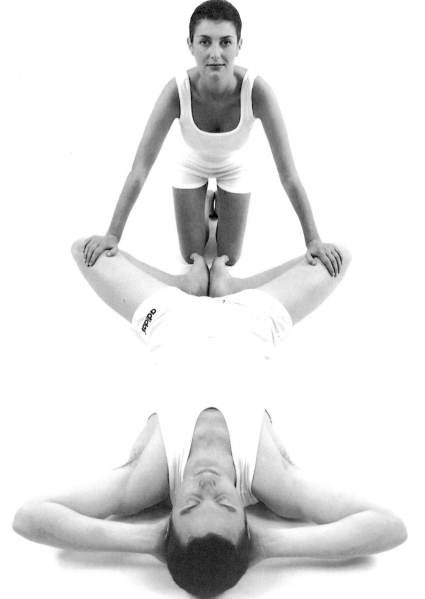

I Lie on the floor and bring your knees up to form a horizontal right angle to your body. Place the soles of your feet together and let your knees come out to the side. Your partner then kneels in front of you and places their hands just above your knees on the inside of the thighs. Then resist against your partner's hands, pushing up for ten seconds while your partner prevents any movement. Stop resisting and allow your partner to ease the knees down a little further. Repeat.

$\mathcal{T}$hese stretches are drawn from Proprioceptive Neuromuscular Facilitation (PNF) techniques which are very effective at developing a full range of movement. PNF techniques work by taking a muscle into a stretch and then tensing up against the resistance offered by your partner for several seconds before relaxing. The muscle worked will often be a little more supple than previously and if repeated three or four times, the stretch will become noticeably deeper and deeper.

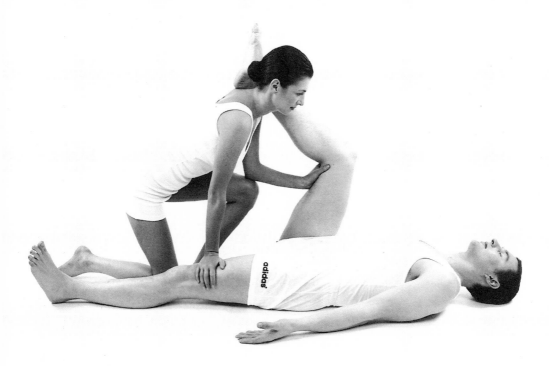

2 This move opens up the hips and thighs. Lying on the floor, bring one leg up. Your partner then puts one hand on the top of the thigh of the straight leg and the other under the knee joint of the raised leg. Resist for a full ten seconds and then relax, while your partner tries to bring the raised leg closer to the chest. Repeat until you feel the muscles softening and becoming more supple.

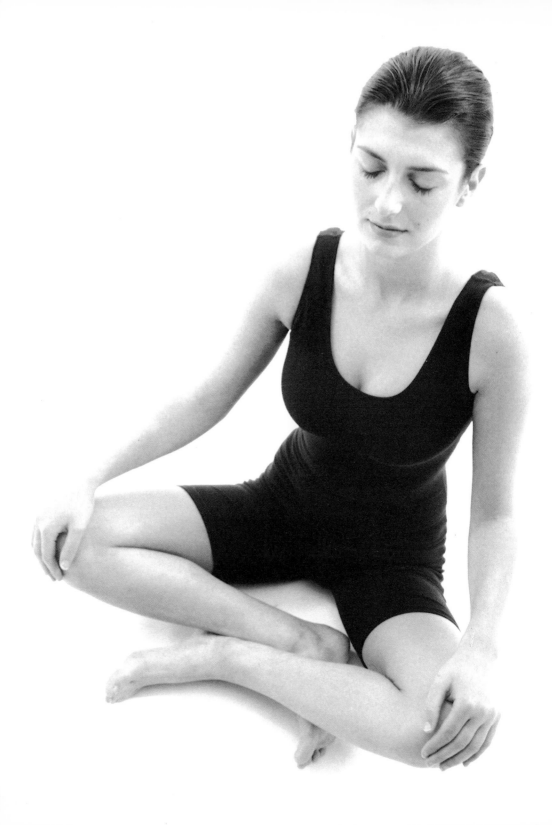

Winding Down

$\mathscr{S}$leep should be an oasis of peace, a tranquil time of rest and regeneration, allowing us to repair our bodies and gather our energies ready for the next day.

But more and more of us are finding it difficult to obtain a restful night's sleep after a busy day, with many unable to stop the same thoughts endlessly cycling in their head, and others drifting fitfully in and out of sleep throughout the night.

With life becoming increasingly pressurized and more demands being made upon our time and energy, it becomes ever more important that we take steps to learn how to relax physically and mentally and let go of everything that has gone on during the day.

Not doing so can have a negative effect on our health over time, with stress and tension building up in our muscles and tissues, over-stimulating our nervous system, depleting our available energy and ageing us needlessly.

So as the day draws to a close, try some of the stretches in this section which are designed to release the cares of the day and prepare you for a restful night ahead. Think of them as physical meditations for mind, body and spirit, aligning and centring you, releasing unwanted tension and worries. Do them regularly enough, and I guarantee you will notice a difference in how you begin to feel. So don't get wound up, wind down instead!

RELEASING THE DAY

I don't know about you but my days are pretty hectic, filled with work projects and business meetings, connecting with friends and family, doing mundane things like shopping and cleaning and – on occasion – even enjoying a splash of romance. Most people lead similar lives, trying to squeeze the demands of work, family, and social life into a 24-hour day. Small wonder, then, that by the end of the day we can be fairly tired and physically tense. Taking time to stretch can not only help us to let go of the day and physically relax us, releasing positive life energy locked within tense muscles, but can also calm us mentally, preparing us for a good night's rest and leaving us looking and feeling rejuvenated the following morning.

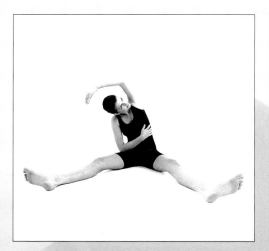

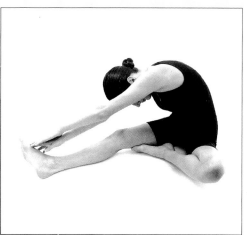

1 Sit down on the floor with your legs wide apart. Look towards your left foot, place your right arm on your ribs and chest and as you breathe in, raise your left arm. Breathe out and lower your left arm in line with the right leg. Repeat on the other side.

2 Then tuck one of your legs into your groin and lean forward along the outstretched leg. Take your time with this and stretch as you breathe out. When you've gone as far as you can, try the other leg.

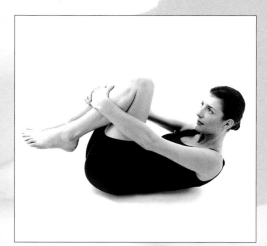

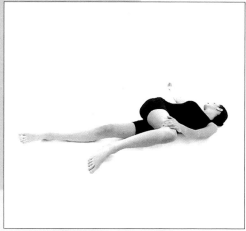

3 Lie on your back and bring both knees up to your chest. By wrapping your arms around them, you can create a deeper stretch along your back. You might find it soothing to rock gently back and forth.

4 Finally, lying on your back, bring your right leg over your left leg and bring it closer to the ground with your left hand. This should create a good stretch along the spine. Balance by repeating with the left leg.

The cares and worries of a full day can rapidly be forgotten by practising some gentle movement or energy work. I really enjoy ending a day with some Tai Chi, which is a Chinese soft martial art, and I'll often throw in some Qi Gong (Chi Gong) energy techniques as well. Combining the two helps to unite the energies of both the earth and the sky and I am left feeling stronger, calmer, lighter, suppler, and with my internal energy flowing more smoothly. So try this mixed routine and let the cares of the day quietly drop away.

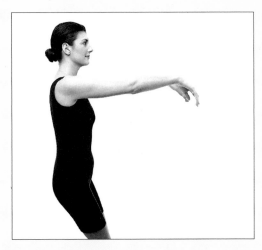

1 Start with your feet together and your hands by your sides. Slowly raise your arms to shoulder height, breathing in as you do so. As your arms become horizontal, bend your knees slightly.

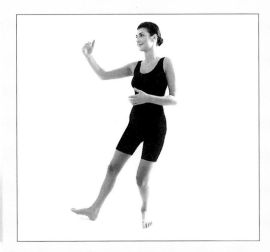

4 Pivot on your right heel and bring your right arm out to the side and your left hand by your chest, and bend slightly to the right. This is an open stance.

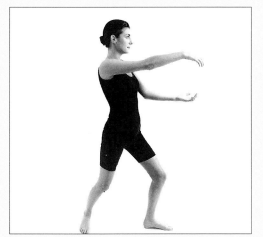

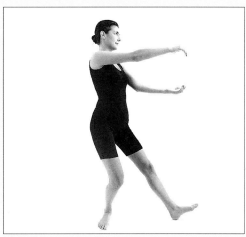

2 Bring your right hand across to the left side, pivoting on your right foot and turning your torso. At the same time allow your left hand to turn palm upwards so that when you have turned fully it looks as if you are cupping a fragile cylinder between your two hands.

3 Then let your left foot come up so that it rests on the heel. Shift your weight on to the back foot and sink your whole body down slightly.

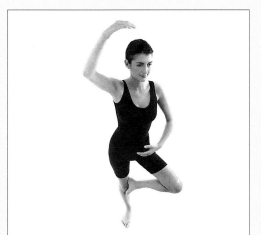

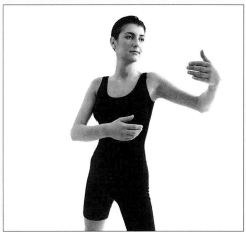

5 Next bring your left foot to the side of your right leg and your right arm above your head. This will test your balancing skills.

6 Bring your left leg down and keep your right arm towards the front of your body, your left hand slightly to the side of you.

I Sit on the floor and cross your legs. Gently rest your hands on your knees and get a sense of how you are sitting. Let the bottom of your spine sink deeper into the floor, keep your head level and imagine your spine elongating to create space between the top and the bottom ends.

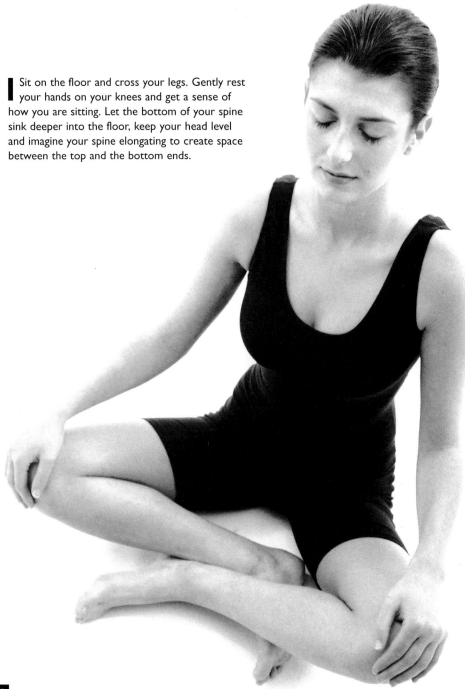

$\mathcal{D}$oing yoga is not always a matter of adopting odd or difficult shapes – some of the most effective poses are also the simplest and most effective for deep relaxing. Here are two of my favourite poses that to help calm and centre me after a busy day. So make sure you have some peace and quiet, the lights are down low, your surroundings warm and comfortable, your clothing light and loose and let's do some evening yoga.

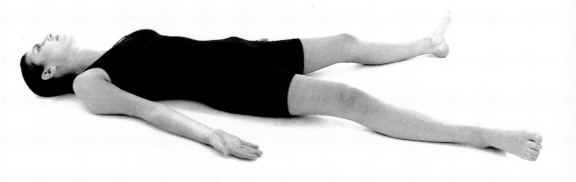

2 Lie on your back and spread your feet widely apart. Place your hands palms up about 6 inches (15cm) away from your sides, and begin to slowly turn your limbs out and then back in. Turn your head from side to side and let it slowly come back to the centre. Imagine that you are being pulled from the legs, creating space in the knee joints and the hips, and that your head is being pulled from your shoulders, releasing tension in the neck. Allow gravity to bring you closer to the ground, breathe from your belly and with each breath feel yourself melt further into the floor.

INFINITY DANCE

The Infinity Dance honours the freshness and potential creativity which exists in every day. Every time it is performed it is unique and personal, and the more times it is experienced the more opportunities arise for allowing creativity in our lives.

From the outside, this may not look very much like the sort of stretching you may be familiar with since it doesn't involve targeting specific muscles or adopting any one specific posture. Rather, it is about listening and feeling – a very personal form of stretching where your body has an opportunity to have its say and do what it needs to.

Find a comfortable position from which to start. Then, with the slowest movements and with full awareness, allow yourself to start moving in whatever way you like. The important thing is not to hurry but to track the movements as they flow into one another, dancing to your own inner music.

The most challenging aspect of this exercise is trust. Trusting what you feel, trusting that you don't have to know everything in advance, that your body knows what to do and can be trusted to do what it needs. So if you feel like making any sound, assuming any shape, say yes and just do it.

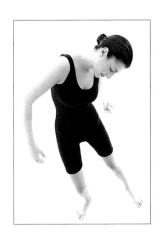

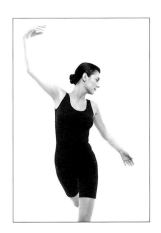

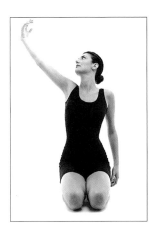

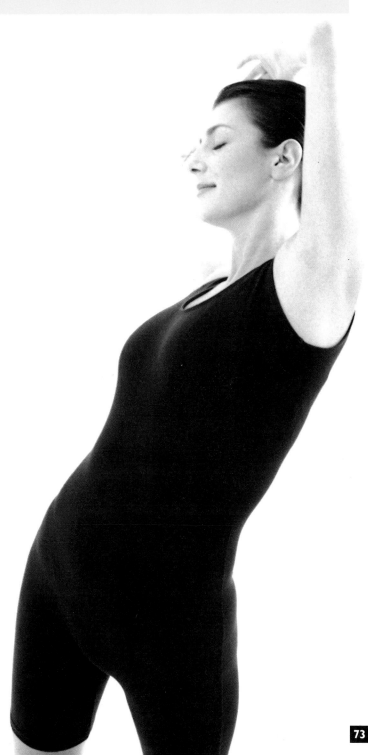

L E T T I N G   I T   A L L   G O

*W*inding down with another person can be a great way of spending quality time together, a way of quietly sharing the end of the evening. Here are some suggestions which can allow your body to let go on a deep level all the stresses and strains of a hectic day. The important thing for the person helping to create the release is that they stay relaxed and calm in their attitude yet focused and alert throughout. This will help them to 'listen' and become aware of small changes in their partner's body as they work.

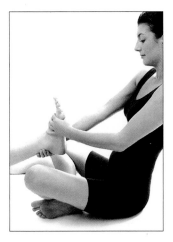

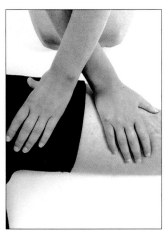

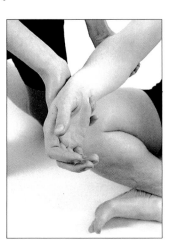

1 Ask your partner to lie on their back and then sit cross-legged in front of their feet. Take one of their feet, support it with both hands and gently lean back until you feel a subtle stretch right up into the top of the leg which, if you are very patient, will open and release further. Change legs and repeat.

2 Cross your hands on your partner's thigh and stretch outwards with both hands. When you've taken the area into a maximum stretch, wait there for a couple of minutes and see if you can detect small releases under your hands as the area slowly opens up.

3 Take your partner's hand and arm. After a few moments you may begin to notice some very small movements occurring spontaneously in either part. The important thing is to follow the movements and allow the body part to unwind in its own time. With practice you'll soon be able to detect the most subtle movements and releases.

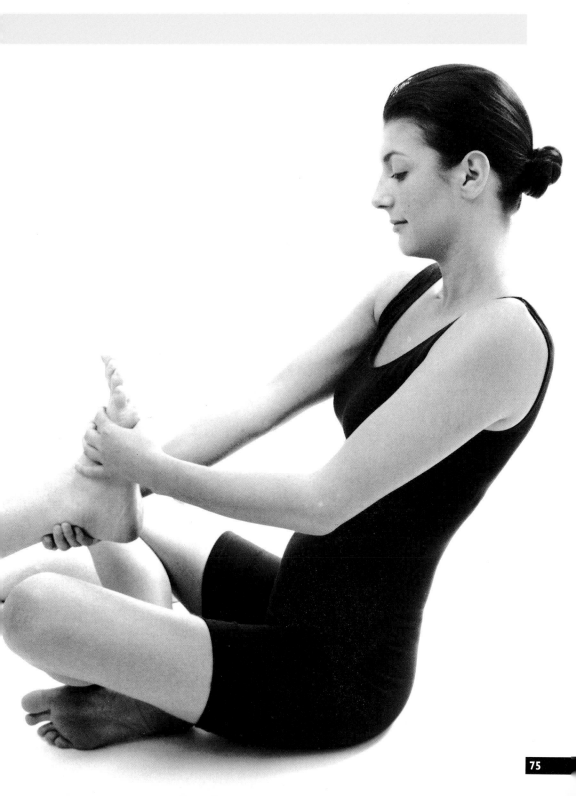

*P*lacing your body in the hands of another individual always brings up questions of trust. No matter how long we may have known someone, it is always surprising to see how inhibited we are about allowing ourselves to relax physically and receive support from another.

These are two of my favourite class exercises. Gentle yet powerful, they will help you to become aware of the secret places in your body where you hold tension and allow you to release this in a safe way, creating a deep sense of calm and physical openness.

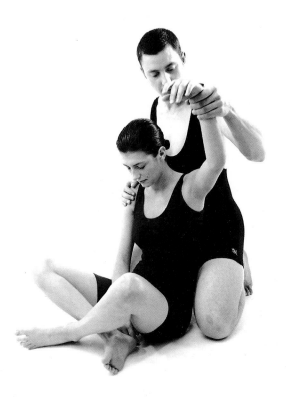

1 Rag doll

Kneel behind your partner who is sitting on the floor and encourage them to lean against you and soften their muscles, going floppy or limp like a rag doll so that you can move their body in any direction. This needs a lot of sensitivity on your part and you should aim to provide a sense of support and security at all times. If any part of your partner's body begins to stiffen or resist movement, softly draw their attention to it and encourage them to continue breathing and let go when appropriate.

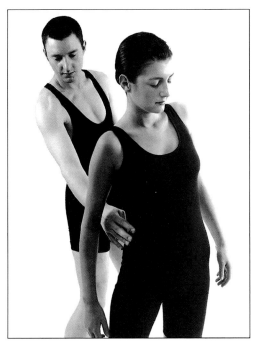

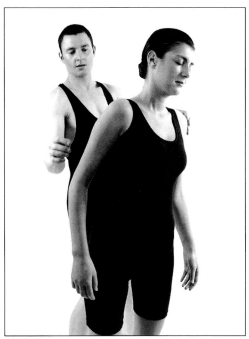

2 Seaweed

Imagine you are a piece of seaweed rooted to the sea floor. Your feet cannot move, but the rest of your body (arms, head, knees, hips and so forth) are seaweed strands which drift and respond instantly to the ever-changing sea current which is represented by your partner's hands. Close your eyes and where the current touches you, begin to move with the same speed and direction. The secret is to bend and flow with the current without losing your secure footing: simultaneously strong yet supple.

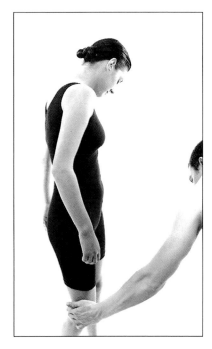

For the person who is the sea current this exercise is about being creative. Try different types of touch; different speeds; different parts and angles of the body. As the session progresses the seaweed should soften and become more fluid and at the end of the session internally that person should feel very different – much calmer, centred, lighter, looser.

Stretching

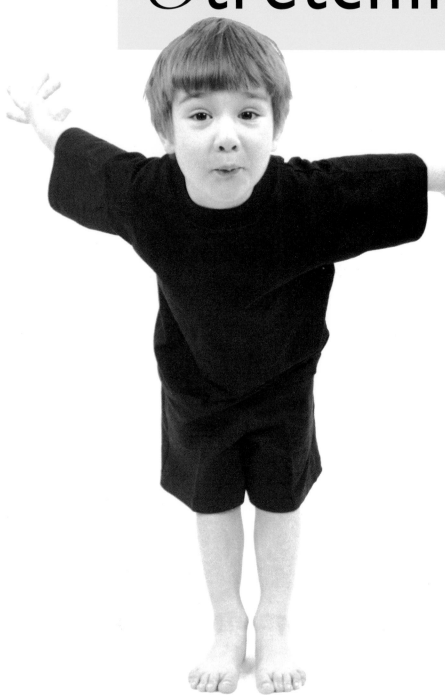

With Innocents

*O*ne of the joys of being a child is the sense of endless energy and possessing a body full of physical possibility and freedom.

It truly is one of the pleasures of life to discover what it feels like to run with the wind in your hair for the first time, or to use not just your hands and feet but your entire body to climb an impossibly large tree. Early experiences like these are invaluable in helping children enjoy their bodies and encouraging them to explore fully their physical potential. In addition, considerable evidence suggests that movement or physical activity, particularly during early childhood, helps to stimulate mental development.

However, with a society that is becoming increasingly sedentary, children today are generally much less active than in previous generations, and are likely to be more familiar with the family video or computer entertainment system than with the potential of their own bodies. If instead they learn to be playful with their bodies and enjoy movement from an early age, this can often help them remain healthy and flexible as they develop into adults.

Often all that is needed from you is a little encouragement to ignite their enthusiasm for movement. They'll enjoy mimicking you, but an added bonus will be the fun they'll have watching you. Naturally supple in their early years, children usually have the edge on adults when it comes to stretching. So be prepared to laugh and be laughed at – because that's what happens when you stretch with innocents.

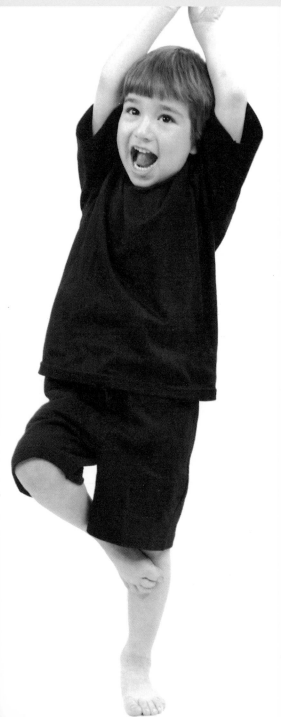

A child's imagination is tremendously powerful. Objects or events which to an adult seem quite solid and real are in the eyes of a child fluid and magical, full of endless possibility. With less sense of a fixed self than an adult, children can assume the identity of a teacup or evil earth-invading alien with surprising ease.

In learning how to become what they imagine, children develop skills which help them to understand the world and people around them. Becoming a mountain is far and away a more powerful experience than just thinking about one. So feel free to use these poses as a springboard to other ideas and happy travels!

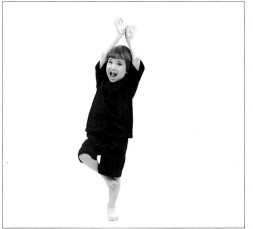

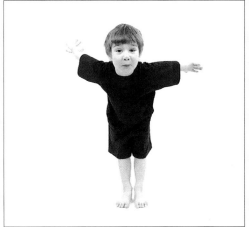

1 Slowly place one foot on the inside of the other leg. It might be a little tricky to keep your balance, but if you think of your toes as roots, breathe slowly and imagine yourself as a strong tree, this might make it a little easier. Then bring your arms out above your head and spread them out like branches of a tree.

2 What does it feel like to be a mountain? Start with both feet together and feel your weight sinking into the floor. Standing straight, gently stretch yourself upwards so that you feel very tall and heavy at the same time. See how slowly you can breathe.

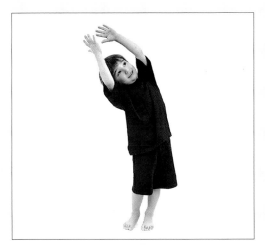

3 Raise your hands right up and imagine touching a rainbow just above your head. As you stretch to touch the right side of the rainbow, let your hips move to the left. This creates a stretch from the wrist to the hip. Repeat on the left.

4 Stretch your arms behind you so they look like the wings of a plane. Then bend forwards slightly and imagine yourself like the wind. How would that feel? How blows the wind?

FUNNY SHAPES

Modern society encourages three basic body positions: standing, sitting, and lying down. However, the body is capable of hundreds of different positions which are discovered and rediscovered many times during childhood, though as we get older these can become a distant memory.

Children love discovering what their bodies can do, and will probably have several favourite positions that they've worked out for themselves. However, you can enlarge their repertoire by showing them a couple of these poses and see what names they come up with. Afterwards, let them use their imagination to create new and vividly named poses.

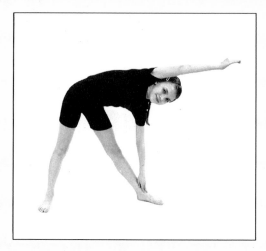

With feet well apart, left foot pointing to the left, raise your left arm so that it is parallel with your shoulder and bring your right arm straight up by the side of your head. Inhale and as you breathe out, bend slightly forward and to the left. Allow your left hand to slide down the leg as far as it can.

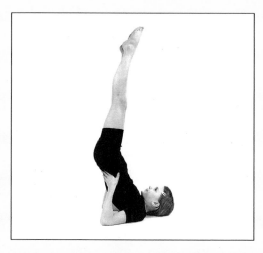

4 Lie face up on the floor with feet together and hands palms down by your sides. Raise your legs, keeping them straight, then bring your hips up and allow your legs to go slightly past your head and push your legs up straight.

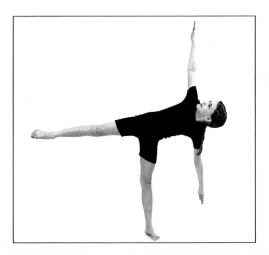

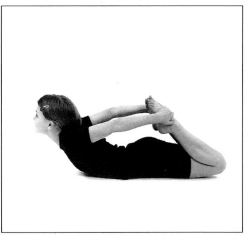

2 Stand with feet apart and arms stretched out to the side. Put your weight on to the left leg and balance on it. Then bend your body to the left, bringing the right hand up vertically, and hold.

3 Lie face downwards with your legs apart. Breathe in and bend your knees. Reach behind and clasp your ankles and breathe out. Breathing in, lift your head and chest and at the same time, lift both your knees off the floor so that you form a bow. Breathe slowly and release.

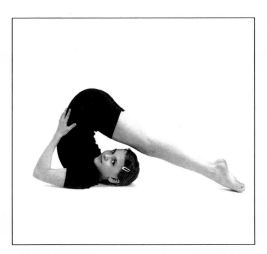

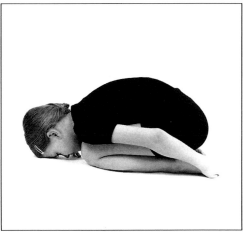

5 If you allow your feet to go over and touch the floor, you'll find you are now in a position traditionally called the plough.

6 The child's pose is a good counterbalancing stretch after the shoulder stand or plough. Stay in this position for a few moments, enjoying a sense of calm and quiet.

𝒞hildren are natural yogis. In exploring the various shapes they can make with their bodies they often stumble across classic yoga poses thousands of years old, many of which were originally inspired by the animal kingdom.

By teaching them a few more poses, you can also turn them into budding wildlife explorers. One game you can play is to show them a particular animal pose and get them to copy it and guess which animal it is. If they get it right, encourage them to make some sounds associated with that animal and really become that creature.

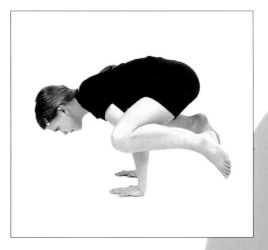

1 Squat down and place your arms between your knees. Make sure your palms are flat and hands are facing forwards. Then push your elbows out so that your knees can rest on the back of the arms. Look ahead, breathe in and lift your toes up, placing the weight into your hands. Breathe out.

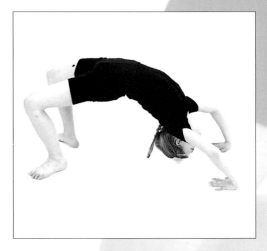

4 Lie on your back and bring your feet near your bottom so that your knees are pointing up. Then arch your arms and place your hands palms down on the floor. Push up from your bottom and gradually straighten your arms until you come into the crab position.

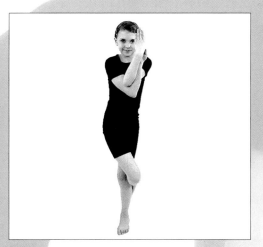

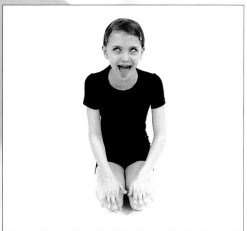

2 The eagle is quite a challenge. Place your weight on to your left leg and bend it slightly, then wrap your right leg around it. Place your right forearm in front of your face and wrap your left arm around it. Squeeze your limbs tight and hold for as long as possible.

3 This is a really silly pose: kids will love it. Sit back on your heels and place your hands on your knees with the fingers splayed out. Breathe in, lean forward slightly, breathe out through your mouth, stretch your tongue out and down, really stretch your fingers, roll your eyeballs up and roar loudly like a lion.

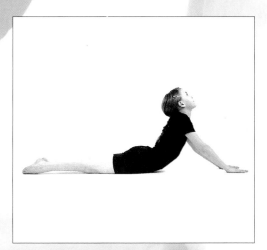

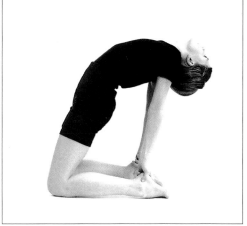

5 Lie on your tummy, palms in front of you. Breathe in and raise your head and shoulders. Tilt your head back and as you breathe out, use your hands to continue to push your trunk away from the floor to become a cobra.

6 Now try the camel. Kneel on the floor with both knees close together and your feet flat on the floor. Then stretch away from the hips, curve your back, bring your head back. Grasp both heels with your hands and breathe.

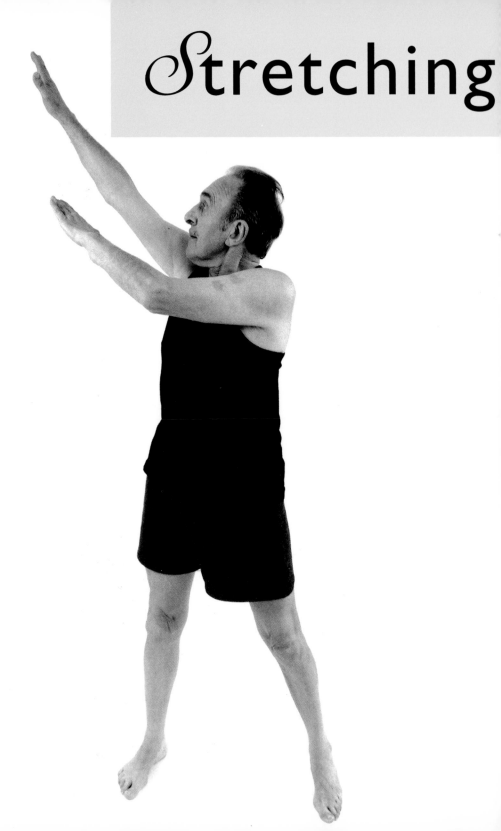

Stretching

With Wisdom

One of the major factors which will determine how you age is movement. Movement oils the body, toning the muscles, strengthening the bones, lubricating the tissues and stimulating the nerves.

The body is extremely adaptable and responsive and if we use it consistently and respectfully throughout our lives, it will answer our needs and respond accordingly. However, if we decide not to use it, the miracle of movement that is flesh and bone can slowly seize up and rather than flowing freely and easily throughout our entire body, our life-force – our energy – can become trapped in stiff muscles and neglected joints.

In the Far East, people generally keep active throughout the course of their lives, often retaining their youthfulness, grace and vitality as they grow older, so that on many occasions they can appear up to 20 years younger than their actual age. There is a general view that every year lived is another step towards elderhood, vitality and wisdom. This contrasts strongly with the West, where the general belief is that growing older will result not in more life, but in less; not in strength, but in weakness; not in health, but in infirmity; not in a blooming of wisdom but a fading of faculties.

Including stretching in your daily routine can be a positive step and will help keep your body strong and supple, your mind active and young, and your spirit filled with grace as you enter your later years as an elder.

STANDING TALL

*O*ur bodies need gravity. In its absence, as astronauts who have spent a long time in space have discovered, they start to deteriorate, with bones softening and muscles wasting away without any force to work against. Gravity enables us to become physically strong as we develop and helps connect and root us to the earth. However, as we get older it can begin to exert a less positive influence, compressing our joints, pulling us closer to the earth, encouraging us to shrink into our bodies and ageing us prematurely.

Yet the earth's gravity is not the only force at play here: we are also subtly pulled by the sky and the stars beyond. We can strike a balance within our own bodies by ensuring that our muscles are relaxed, our tissues loose and our joints free with space to move. Doing so will enable us to stand tall to experience the freedom and wonder in each and every day.

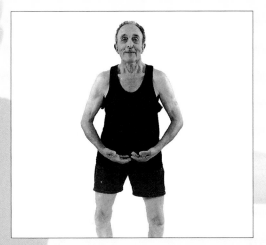

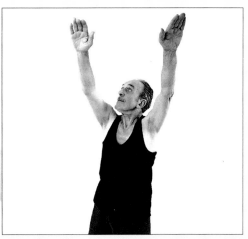

1 Stand with your knees slightly bent and allow the earth to support your weight fully. Breathe from your abdomen, relax your shoulders and imagine a hook from the sky connecting to your head, gently pulling upwards.

2 Then imagine that your hands have become eagles soaring in the sky above. Move them in circles and allow that movement to be echoed in your hips and knees.

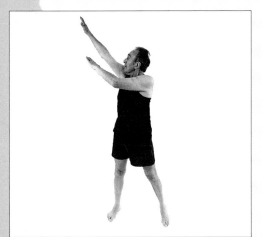

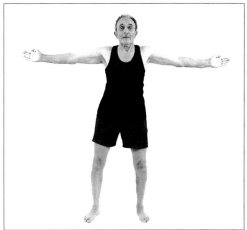

3 Next sweep with both hands to your right and then to the other side, using gravity to give you a bit of speed and momentum. Breathe in as you sweep up and breathe out as the arms come down.

4 Finally stand with your legs apart, your weight sinking firmly into the ground. Stretch your arms out to the side as far as they can go and see if you can feel the fingertips stretch and your whole arm become longer. Keep your head loose and the spine gently stretched. How does this feel?

*W*ithin many traditional cultures the breath is considered sacred, with an importance equalling that of food for the wellbeing of the individual. With each breath life-giving oxygen is drawn into every part of the body and subtle energy from the environment is absorbed to help strengthen the immune system and maintain health. In these societies, many breathing techniques have been developed to maximize the quantity and quality of the air breathed.

Good breathing brings more oxygen to the brain, expels toxins, improves our energy levels and helps to make us feel physically and mentally calm and relaxed. So no matter how long you've already been breathing, why not take five minutes to try these exercises and experience a new breath of life?

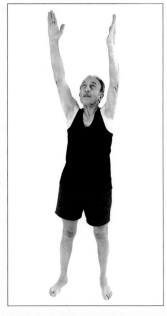

I Slowly raise both arms up to meet above your head. Breathe in from your belly and feel the air expanding in your chest. Bring your hands down slowly, exhaling as you do so, and feel your whole body lengthen when you bring them up again.

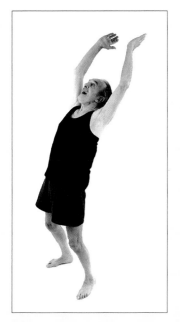

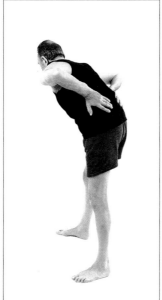

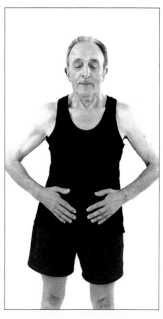

2 Next squeeze your buttocks tight, stretch slightly backwards and expel all your breath out through your mouth with a large AAHHH! sound. You can release a lot of tension and stiffness by making circles with your upper body. Straighten up, lower your arms and repeat three times.

3 Next place your hands by your waist and lower back. Then turn your upper body at an angle to the right and bend slightly to look down. Then allow the upper body to travel to the opposite side in a smooth semi-circle, breathing slowly as you bend forward.

4 Stand with feet apart and hands resting lightly on your abdomen. Take a slow breath through the nose and bring it down into the abdomen, pushing your hands out slightly. Breathe out through your mouth and repeat. See if you can use your imagination to bring breath into every part of your body.

$\mathcal{M}$ovement is the driving force behind life. We express this force with full intensity in our early years, yet as we mature there can be a tendency to become less physical, less active. However, not exploring the full potential for movement contained within our bodies can mean that muscles and tissues become stiff and compressed, which in turn can cause a slowing and stagnation of our energy and a spiral towards even more inactivity, even less life.

However, older people who keep active often find that constant, varying movement brings with it physical and mental freedom, high levels of energy, a great sense of vitality and zest for life. So the choice is yours. Do you want to wear a blindfold in front of a beautiful sunset, or do you want to appreciate every hue and then stay up to welcome the sunrise too?

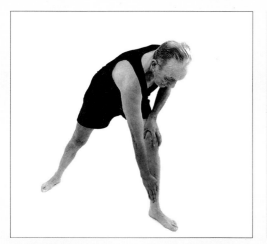

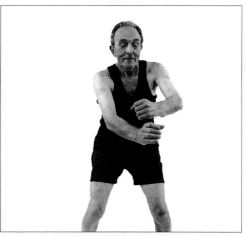

1 Stand with your legs well apart. Place your left hand on the left knee and with your right hand lean forward to touch your left ankle or foot. Shift your weight across and swop hands to repeat on the other side.

2 Now imagine you are stirring a huge cauldron with a big spoon in your hands. Let your whole body follow the movement of your hands.

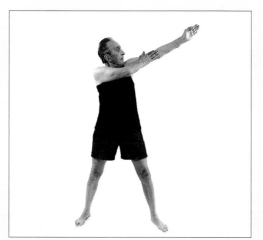

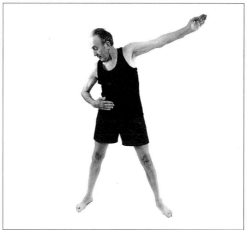

3 Then swing your arms from side to side and let your right hand sweep along the left arm and then as you swing to the other side let the left hand sweep along the right arm.

4 Next include a brushstroke which goes from the palm of the outstretched hand, along the arm, diagonally across the body and finally down the front of the opposite thigh. Let a rhythm emerge and repeat on the other side.

APPENDIX

There may be times when one part of your body needs some extra flexibility. Perhaps, like most people, you'd like your back to be a little more loose and supple. You'll find a wide choice of both individual and partner stretches to choose from in the back section. Alternatively, you might want to develop an overall suppleness in your body. If so, why not try some of the stretches in the whole body section?

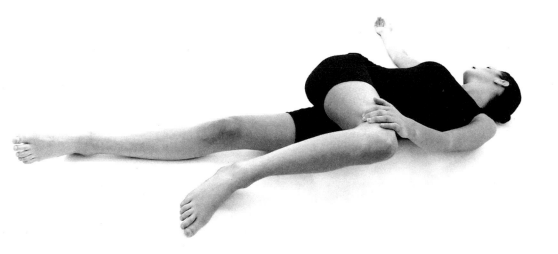

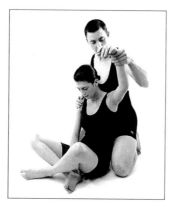

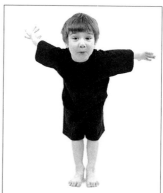

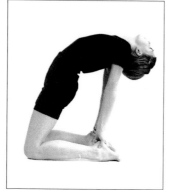

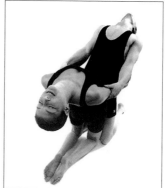